LEARNING TO PLAY GOD

The Coming of Age of a Young Doctor

Robert Marion, M.D.

FAWCETT CREST • NEW YORK

A Fawcett Crest Book
Published by Ballantine Books
Copyright © 1991 by Robert Marion, M.D.

Portions of this book appeared in somewhat different form in *The Journal of the American Medical Association*, *New York Doctor*, and *The Einstein Quarterly*.

Library of Congress Catalog Card Number: 91-14517

ISBN 0-449-22192-X

This edition published by arrangement with Addison-Wesley Publishing Company, Inc.

Printed in Canada

First Ballantine Books Edition: April 1993

More praise for
Dr. Robert Marion and
LEARNING TO PLAY GOD

To Lewis Fraad, M.D.
(1907–1990)
Pediatrician, medical educator,
human being

He who teaches a child is
as if he had created it.
                    —*The Talmud*

Contents

Part III: Residency

Prologue

The applicant, a senior at Dartmouth College, had perched himself so precariously on the edge of my office couch that I got the feeling he was preparing to bolt out of the room at any moment. Sitting like that, dressed in his dark gray pinstriped suit, white oxford shirt, and blue-and-white striped tie, an outfit that was apparently the unofficial uniform of all male medical school applicants, the student seemed extremely uncomfortable during the first twenty minutes or so of the interview.

But there was no reason for the young man to feel uncomfortable: he was clearly a winner. In addition to having an impressive undergraduate grade point average from a prestigious college and excellent scores on all sections of the Medical College Aptitude Test, the letters of recommendation he'd received from his professors at Dartmouth were outstanding. And if all this wasn't enough, during the past few summers the applicant had done extensive volunteer work at a hospice in his native New Jersey, caring for terminally ill cancer patients, and his folder contained glowing testimonials from three separate patients who swore that their last days had been touched and improved by the presence of this wonderful young man. No, this applicant didn't need to worry; he was a shoo-in for acceptance at our medical school. All he had to do was make it through the interview without coming off as a complete social misfit.

But coming off as a complete social misfit seemed exactly what he was determined to do. Though I tried to get him to relax by asking a series of what I considered nonthreatening, low-pressure questions about his background, he grew increasingly nervous and distressed, picking intensely at the cuticle of his left thumbnail, biting repeatedly on his lower lip, and breathing rapidly. I could not engage him in an extended conversation; he answered my questions with one- or two-word responses, little more than grunts really, and I was becoming concerned that either the secretaries in the admissions office had mistakenly handed me the wrong applicant's folder before the interview had begun or, even worse, this young man of sterling credentials was about to have a psychotic break right before my eyes.

But thankfully, things changed for the better when I finally got around to asking him The Question. In retrospect, I guess he must have thought I was trying to trick him with all those other questions, trying to get him to trip up and say something potentially damaging that would immediately disqualify him from consideration for a place in our medical school class, and so he'd kept up his guard and maintained a psychological distance. But now, at long last, we had gotten down to the only area of substance which had to be covered in a medical school interview. All his nervousness and distress immediately melted away when I said these words:

"So tell me: why is it that you've decided to become a doctor?"

Instantly, he sat back on the couch, and his breathing returned to a more normal rate; he stopped picking at his nail and biting his lower lip, and for the first time since he'd entered my office, his eyes met mine. "I've wanted to be a doctor for as long as I can remember," he began, speaking freely, with genuine emotion. "I've loved science ever since I was a little kid; it's always been my strongest subject in school. And I want to do something with my life to help others, to try to make the world a better place to live. As far as I can see, a career in medicine is the best way to combine these two interests.''

With the pressure off, we spent the next twenty minutes talking calmly. He told me what he imagined life would be like after he became a physician; we discussed the type of medicine he had considered practicing and where he'd like to live. No more during the course of the interview did the young man appear tentative, or nervous, or distressed. Because he had finished it so well, I decided to dismiss the concerns I'd had about him during the first half of the interview as nothing more than nervousness, something that's acceptable in any applicant. And less than a month after the interview, that senior from Dartmouth received a letter in the mail offering him a place in the first-year class of our medical school beginning the following September.

During the three years that I have been a member of the admissions committee at our medical school, I've interviewed well over a hundred applicants. Although these candidates have descended on the Bronx from very different backgrounds, representing both sexes in fairly equal numbers and coming from an assortment of nationalities and races, nearly all of them have had two things in common. First, the vast majority of them have shown up in my office's waiting room looking well groomed and all similarly dressed in conservative clothing. Not once during interview season has an applicant appeared at my door dressed in purple madras pants, or a dashiki in the colors of the flag of the African National Congress, or with hair dyed orange and worn in a Mohawk. All have chosen to conform to the medical school-applicant ''look.''

The second feature these applicants have shared is far more significant than the outfits they chose to wear to their interviews. Well over 90 percent of them have told me, with what seemed like genuine feeling, that their motivation to seek a career in medicine is the same as that expressed by the student from Dartmouth: they want to advance scientific knowledge, and they want to do something with their lives that will help their fellow man; after careful consideration, it struck them that medicine was the perfect way to combine these two aspirations.

And that's terrific. The desire to help one's fellow man should be a major driving force at the heart of a young person's decision to seek a career in medicine. A sincere desire to aid humanity, to help the infirm, to give comfort to those who are in pain is a trait that society should expect from its physicians. Doctors have to care greatly *about* their patients, not just for them; they must be concerned about the state of patients' minds and spirits as well as about the ills that afflict their bodies. Medical educators should foster the idealism that brings applicants to medical school in the first place, allowing it to grow and ultimately blossom into true humanism.

But is this happening? Does the early idealism of medical students thrive during the grueling training young doctors undergo in medical school and during their internships and residencies? Is the system that trains our physicians, which has been in place for over a hundred years now, geared toward nurturing those features that society should demand in its doctors, while weeding out other, negative features? I have written this book to try to answer these questions.

The stories told in this volume are all true. Although the names of patients, doctors, other staff members, and even some hospitals have been changed in order to preserve anonymity as much as possible, every event chronicled here actually occurred to me or my colleagues during our medical training. Written at the time of the events' occurrence or reconstructed later from notes kept in a journal, the stories are arranged chronologically, from the day I started medical school through the end of my residency. From these vignettes, which should be considered as single frames on a reel, a fairly realistic motion picture emerges, documenting what it's like to train as a physician in the United States in the latter half of the twentieth century.

* * *

This book could not have been written without the assistance and inspiration of the teachers who helped me make it through the years that are spanned here. There would have been no beginning had it not been for Stephen Lazar, Ed.D. and Sasha Englard, Ph.D., both of whom had faith in me, and went out on a limb to help a guy who didn't have terrific credentials. There would have been no story had it not been for my medical school adviser, Tom Daley, M.D., and for my very close friends, Andy Mezey, M.D., Steve Shelov, M.D., and Michael Cohen, M.D., each of whom rescued me from the brink of disaster on more than one occasion. Most important, I owe a tremendous debt of gratitude to Lewis Fraad, M.D., pediatrician and medical educator, who touched the lives of thousands of physicians in all medical specialties who trained in the New York area, and to whose memory this book is dedicated.

I'd also like to acknowledge the following persons: Diana Finch, my literary agent, who, once again, always seems to be there for me when I need her most; Johanna van Hise, Carolyn Savarese, Nancy Fish, and Jane Isay, my friends at Addison-Wesley; and Nancy Miller, my editor, who with her husband, Stephen Kling, are my best friends in the world. And finally, I'd like to thank Beth for her love and understanding, and Isadora, Davida, and Jonah for allowing me occasional access to the computer.

PART I

Medical School

1

How I Got Here

**Schweitzer School of Medicine
orientation, August 29, 1974**

By the time I entered at a few minutes before nine, the auditorium was nearly full; 150 or so well-rested, seemingly happy but also obviously nervous souls were already seated in the room, talking anxiously with their new classmates sitting beside them, passing the time until the program was scheduled to begin. Taking one of the few empty seats near the rear of the room, I couldn't help smiling. As the seconds passed, that small smile gradually blossomed into the kind of broad, full-faced grin that, unprovoked, might be expected to be seen only on the face of a crazy person. But I wasn't crazy. I had a perfectly valid reason to be ecstatic. After all the ups and downs of the past few years, after all the disappointing interviews and letters of rejection from admissions committees, after the failed efforts of friends and acquaintances and my ultimate decision to leave the country in order to get an education, I had at last gotten the chance to be a medical student at the Albert Schweitzer School of Medicine in New York.

When the remainder of the class had filed in and silently filled all the empty seats, Dr. Matthews, the dean of the medical school, stepped to the podium at the front of the room and began his welcoming remarks. He spoke

3

for nearly half an hour, and his comments were followed
by an entire orientation program, but I lost the thread
almost immediately; I couldn't concentrate on what anyone was saying. Instead, my thoughts kept drifting off,
back to the year before. Rather than sitting in an anonymous, unnumbered chair in this relative palace of an auditorium that served as the permanent lecture hall for the
first-year class at the Albert Schweitzer School of Medicine in the Bronx, New York, I thought back to the year
before—to my assigned seat, number 68, in the small,
dingy, poorly maintained auditorium in which lectures
were delivered to the preregistration class at the Royal
College of Surgeons in Dublin, Ireland. Although less
than a year had passed since I'd first sat in that seat, I
felt as though all my experiences as a preregistration student had occurred in a completely separate lifetime.

For most young people who seek a career in medicine,
the path taken from start to finish is fairly straightforward
and simple. The process usually goes something like this:
during the senior year of college, after meeting with a
professional-school adviser, the student completes and
mails applications to a carefully selected group of medical schools around the country; after reviewing the applications, the admissions committees at some of those
schools schedule interviews with the student; then, during the course of a forty-five-minute meeting, the interviewer, usually a middle-level faculty member at the
school, decides whether, in his or her opinion, the applicant, after seven or eight years of training, will have
what is needed to be a good physician. If the interviewer's decision is positive, the student will receive an acceptance letter in the mail a few weeks after the
interview—and will spend much of the remainder of the
senior year of college floating on air. If the decision is
negative, a formal rejection letter will be sent. In the vast
majority of cases, at least one of the schools to which
the student has applied will grace him or her with one of
those acceptance letters, and, after graduating from col-

lege, the student will spend the next four years studying medicine in the classroom, the laboratory, and on the wards of the school's affiliated hospitals.

But the path I took from college to medical school was somewhat different from the journey taken by most would-be physicians. My path took me to Ireland, to seat number 68 in the preregistration-year lecture hall.

Standing at the curb, trying to cross St. Stephen's Green as the seconds ticked away, I realized it was only a matter of time before my number would finally be up. Each day, five minutes before the preregistration lecture was scheduled to begin, the attendance officer would come by with his master seating chart to mark off those who were absent. Getting to class before the attendance officer was thus very important, but I was sure that sooner or later, this early in the morning, with the pressure on and my mind not yet fully awake, the day would come when I'd instinctively look to the left, the way I'd been taught to cross busy streets as a child growing up in New York—I'd look to the left and see that the road was clear, and I'd hurriedly step off into the street, only to get creamed by a Guinness delivery truck, or a Dublin city bus, or if I happened to be very lucky, a Morris Mini, any of which might be approaching, perfectly properly, from the right. I was certain that some such catastrophe was bound to happen sometime during the six years I planned to be a medical student in Ireland. But it didn't happen that morning: I did indeed make it to the other side of St. Stephen's Green. Stepping up my pace, I entered the main building of Surgeons by the side entrance and, now nearly running, hurriedly sat down, seconds before the attendance officer entered the classroom.

Attendance at preregistration classes was mandatory. In order to qualify to take the final exams in biology, chemistry, and physics, the three premedical sciences that composed the course work for the preregistration year, we students had to attend at least 80 percent of all scheduled lectures and laboratories. And if we didn't sit for, and pass, those final exams, we wouldn't be permitted to go on to Med-I, the first full year of medical school. So, as the attendance officer left, passing Professor Elliot, the biology teacher who was then entering the hall to begin that day's lecture, I settled down in my seat and tried my best to pay attention.

Although the three courses that made up preregistration year were supposed to be academically equivalent to those of introductory science courses offered to college freshmen back home, they were actually taught at a much lower level, closer to that in an American high school, and sometimes even to junior high school standards. Because one third of my classmates at Surgeons came from countries where English was not the native tongue, in order to make sure these students had at least a fighting chance of keeping up with the class's Irish, English, and American students, the professors covered the material very slowly, repeating sentences over and over again, creating a weirdly scientific, soporific litany.

There were twelve of us Americans in the preregistration class, and each had come to Dublin for the same reason: over the course of the previous few years we had received dozens of rejection letters from American medical schools which made it crystal clear that, because of poor grades, or inadequate scores on the Medical College Aptitude Test, or letters of recommendation that failed to mention our ability to walk on water, we'd never be able to cut it as physicians. These rejection letters had forced us to accept the fact that we weren't going to be given the opportunity to become doctors in the United States. They had spelled out that a decision had to be made, a decision either to abandon our dreams of becoming physicians and pursue other careers, or to abandon our homes and go to a foreign country where we might be able to get a medical education. Faced with these two options, each of the twelve of us had chosen the latter. We had come to Ireland as a last resort; it was either succeed here, or forever live with our failure.

But in spite of the disappointments we had experienced and the dejection we all felt, we knew damned well that we were the lucky ones: our school, the Royal College of Surgeons in Ireland, was the only medical school in the British Isles which even considered applicants from the United States. Most of the other American citizens who'd found themselves in our predicament had wound up attending schools in Mexico, Italy, or Belgium, having to learn the complicated and relatively foreign concepts of biochemistry, physiology, and pathology in complicated and wholly foreign languages. So when each of us—college graduates, a few with master's degrees in biology—had been denied exemption from the high school–level science courses that composed the preregistration year, no one complained. None of us wanted to get thrown out of school.

I hadn't even heard of Surgeons until March of that year, six months prior to beginning classes. Before then I'd spent most of my time hoping and praying that the message Dr. Black, the zoologist who was the chairman of the professional-school advisory committee at my college, had given me at the start of that academic year would prove to be wrong. Back in September, Dr. Black had called me into his office and, very solemnly, informed me that, after carefully reviewing my records and letters of recommendation, he and the other members of the committee had come to the conclusion that I didn't have a snowball's chance in hell of getting into medical school. "The competition's just too much," he told me before launching into a discussion of what he called my options, including applying to dental school ("where the competition isn't as rough") and graduate schools in biology. What Dr. Black told me made sense, but I wouldn't listen. I had my mind and heart set on becoming a doctor, and with just a little divine intervention I was almost positive I could make it.

Naively, I hadn't thought of myself as a typical medical school applicant. Although it was true I'd screwed around in college, attaining only a B-plus grade point average (at a time when most successful applicants to medical school had at least an A-minus), I believed I had a lot of other things going for me. For one, there was my brother, Les. Then an intern in Washington, D.C., Les had graduated from Tulane University's School of Medicine in New Orleans just the year before. He'd done exceedingly well, having been elected president of his class and serving as a student representative on the school's admissions committee. He'd even been on a first-name basis with the chairman of that committee. Surely, in spite of my mediocre record, my brother's pull at Tulane would be more than enough to put me over the top.

And then there was Andy Lipman, whose family had lived in the house next door to ours when I was growing up and who had gone on to become assistant dean at the Albert Schweitzer School of Medicine. Although Andy and I had had little contact during my childhood I was sure that, in a pinch, he could be counted on to put in a good word. So all in all I wasn't that worried. I wasn't worried, that is, until January, when the rejection letters started pouring in.

Rejection letters are easy to spot in the mail. Painfully thin, the envelopes contain just a single sheet of stationery: "After careful consideration of your application," the letters all read, "we regret to inform you that we cannot offer you a place in our medical school class." Regardless of the reasons listed for the rejection, my reaction to these letters was always the same: first a queasiness would develop in the pit of my stomach, then an ache would begin in the front of my head, followed finally by the feeling that I'd had the wind knocked out of me. It got so bad that by February the queasiness began almost as soon as I saw the mailman coming down the street.

The letters came from everywhere, arriving one or two a day. At first they hadn't bothered me much; I'd never really expected to get into Creighton University, or the University of Chicago. But when the letters started coming from schools in New York State, I became more concerned. And then, at the beginning of February, there was the envelope from the Albert Schweitzer School of Medicine. That one hit particularly hard.

But it wasn't until the afternoon when the thin letter with the return address TULANE AVENUE, NEW ORLEANS, LOUISIANA arrived in early March that I realized Dr. Black and his committee had been right all along. Getting that rejection from my brother's alma mater left me depressed and angry at a system that wouldn't allow me to do the one thing in the world I truly wanted to do, resentful of my classmates with higher averages, with better board scores, with superior letters of recommendation who'd already received at least one fat envelope, and some as many as five or six, packages containing lots of forms and instructions and always including a cover letter that began "We are happy to inform you . . ." At the end of four days of intense despondency after receiving that final rejection, I realized it was time to assess my options.

I carefully examined my motivation and my staying power and, after tormenting myself and those around me for nearly a week, I reached a conclusion: I didn't want to be a dentist; I didn't want to be a graduate student in biology and end up teaching; what I most wanted to do was to be a doctor, and the longer I thought about it, the more I was convinced that I could and would do anything necessary to reach that goal. That's when I began looking into foreign schools.

Attending a foreign medical school is an option chosen by only a small fraction of the would-be physicians who don't get accepted at an American school. Most college students in this predicament elect instead to attend a graduate program in biology or chemistry for a year or two, working hard to get outstanding grades in their graduate-level course work and to improve their MCAT scores so that eventually, with their records shined and gleaming, they can reapply to medical schools, hoping that their previous rejection doesn't hurt their chances. The graduate school route is something of a gamble, but going away from home, leaving friends and family, is a sacrifice most people are not willing to make.

But attending a foreign school was the path I chose to take. I knew that even a few years of graduate school would not guarantee acceptance at an American school, and I didn't think it would be prudent to risk two or more years in the hope that my academic situation would improve drastically. So after a little research, I applied to most of the major foreign schools that accepted American students. When I finally received an acceptance letter, from the huge school in Guadalajara, Mexico, I enrolled in an intensive Spanish course in order to prepare myself for what seemed to be the inevitable. But then in March, through my father's meeting one of his business acquaintances by chance, I heard about Surgeons. This acquaintance, it turned out, had a son who was then a second-year student in Ireland. I promptly wrote to Dublin for an application, and when it arrived I filled it out, sent it back, crossed my fingers, and waited.

The fat envelope with the return address ST. STEPHEN'S GREEN, DUBLIN arrived in early June, and in less than an hour I'd dropped out of the Spanish course. Luck had smiled on me for the first time in months, and my future was bright: I would go to Dublin; I would study there for six years and I would graduate with a degree in medicine.

During the summer before my departure for Dublin, through Andy Lipman, my old neighbor, I got a job working as a technician in the lab of Arthur Rubenstein, a professor of biochemistry at Schweitzer. Although it was only supposed to be a summer job, a way of earning a few bucks and killing the time between graduation from college and the start of the preregistration year at Surgeons, my months of working with Dr. Rubenstein turned out to be much more.

From the beginning, I felt a closeness with Dr. Rubenstein. From early in the morning and into the evening we'd stand side by side at a workbench in his lab, setting up and performing experiments designed to examine the effects of the aging process of the structure of collagen, an important structural protein. We talked while we worked, discussing everything from science to literature to religion. Dr. Rubenstein, who'd been on the Schweitzer faculty since the school's founding in the fifties, was actually interested in the things I had to say; standing beside me, he listened, considered my comments, and responded, treating me as a colleague rather than a lowly student. It was rare that a teacher had treated me in such a way, which gave a tremendous boost to my sagging confidence, and I developed a lasting fondness for him.

As the summer passed, Dr. Rubenstein and I became genuine friends. On a few occasions he invited me to his home to meet his family; he had three daughters, one of whom was then entering her second year as a student at Schweitzer. She and I spent a lot of time talking about medicine and about the kind of life medical students led. The biochemist's interest in me made me work harder in his lab, and, as a result, we accomplished more that summer than either he or I had imagined possible.

No matter how hard I worked in the lab, though, or how close I grew to Dr. Rubenstein and his family, I knew that this experience would soon draw to a close. In early August, I purchased my ticket on Aer Lingus; I'd be leaving for Dublin during the first week of September. One morning shortly before my departure, Dr. Rubenstein called me into his office. "I think you're going to make an excellent physician, Bob," he began; "I truly believe that. I've watched how you've conducted yourself in my lab, how hard you've worked, and how you've related to me and to my family. I've worked at medical schools for a long time, and I've been around a lot of medical students. I think I know what qualities to look for in medical applicants. And you've got those qualities, I'm sure of it."

I blushed and thanked him, but he continued: "I've

made a few phone calls, and unfortunately, it looks like there's nothing I'm going to be able to do to help you this year. But maybe next year. . . . Have you thought about reapplying for next year's class?''

''No,'' I replied. ''I figured there'd be no point. My academic record would be exactly the same as it was this year.''

''That may be so, Bob, but there are two other facts that have to be taken into account this time around. First, you've made the decision to go abroad, and that says a lot about your determination; and second, you've got me on your side, and as you probably know, I'm a member of the admissions committee.''

Until that moment I had had no idea that Dr. Rubenstein was a member of the admissions committee at Schweitzer, but I was sure as hell glad to hear about it. And so, figuring I had nothing to lose but also trying not to be too hopeful, I once again wrote to the American Medical College Application Service for an application form. I spent my last few days before leaving for Ireland filling it out, listing Schweitzer as the only school of medicine to which I'd be applying. I sent the form back, finished my packing, and tried not to think about it anymore.

My interview was scheduled for December 20, the day after I returned to New York from Ireland for Christmas vacation. It was pouring that morning—a sign of good luck, my mother insisted, but to me it only meant that the usually easy thirty-five-minute car trip from my parents' home in Rockland Country to the Schweitzer campus in the Bronx would be treacherous, taking at least twice as long as usual.

When I arrived at the admissions office I was half frozen and soaking wet: my gray suit, bought the year before especially for medical school interviews, was dripping; my hair, cut shorter than usual by a barber in Dublin the day before I came home, was plastered down; my glasses were fogged and water-spotted. Since first impressions are so important, and since this interview was my only chance, I figured I'd blown my opportunity before I even stepped into the interviewer's office.

I was scheduled to be interviewed by a Dr. Harold Chambers, an associate professor in the Department of Medicine. The interview didn't start off on a very positive note: "I see you were rejected here last year," Dr. Chambers began, before even bothering to introduce himself. "Why do you think we should reconsider you now?"

One problem I'd had with interviews in the past was my lack of assertiveness. I'd frequently had trouble being convincing, instead coming across as if I lacked conviction. But that was not the case that morning. "You're right in saying that I was rejected by this medical school last year," I replied firmly. "But I've wanted to be a doctor ever since I was a kid. And I'm going to be a doctor. In fact, I was rejected by over thirty medical schools. Because of those rejections, I decided to go abroad. I'm currently a first-year student at the Royal College of Surgeons in Ireland. So, Dr. Chambers, I'm going to be a doctor; either I'll do it the hard way, in a foreign country, away from my family and friends, or if you'll give me the chance, I'll do it an easier way, here in the Bronx. All I ask is that you give me that chance."

It was the best interview of my life. At the end, when he was saying goodbye and wishing me luck, I asked if, because of my unusual circumstances, it would be possible to get an answer from the admissions committee before I was scheduled to return to Ireland at the beginning of January. Dr. Chambers, shaking my hand, said he'd try his best.

The fat envelope with the return address ALBERT SCHWEITZER SCHOOL OF MEDICINE, MORRIS PARK AVENUE, BRONX, NEW YORK arrived two days after Christmas.

As I sat in my seat near the rear of the auditorium, grinning my foolish grin, I tried to concentrate on what the dean and the other speakers were saying, but it was no use; instead, I thought about all that had happened over the previous twelve months, and I realized again how lucky I was. I'd been given the chance to study medicine at one of the most prestigious medical schools in the entire world. I wasn't going to screw this up; no way was I going to screw this up.

Nearly all American medical schools currently have programs that last for four years. The standard medical curriculum is divided pretty evenly into two separate two-year cycles. During the first cycle, known as the preclinical years, the student learns the basic sciences, the foundation on which clinical training is built. Through lectures, laboratory assignments, and an extensive body of reading material, the first- and second-year medical student learns anatomy, histology, biochemistry, physiology, and pathology; because there is no contact with patients during those first two years, no clinical material to which this science can be related, the material often seems dessicated and empty. Since students come to medical school principally to learn how to care for living, breathing patients, they soon become frustrated and bored. They long to be finished with preclinical work and to get a taste of life in the hospital.

The teaching of the preclinical sciences at the Schweitzer School of Medicine was markedly different from that at the Royal College of Surgeons in Ireland. For one thing, attendance was far from mandatory; there were no assigned seats, no attendance officers, no threats. We students were basically on our own; as long as we showed up for and passed the exams at the end of each course, no one gave a damn whether we even made an appearance on the Schweitzer campus.

In fact, one could get away with not attending classes at all. Since the school's founding, the administration had made it a policy to supply students with a syllabus, a compilation of lecture notes prepared by the faculty members giving the lectures, for every course that was given. All final exams were based on these syllabi, and students could not be held responsible for any material not in the syllabus, even material covered during a lecture or a lab. Simply by studying the syllabus, it was thus possible to pass all courses and get promoted to clinical rotations. And since all preclinical science classes were graded pass/fail, all one had to do was score above a 65 in order to succeed.

Because of the syllabi, the pass/fail system, and the rule governing the material on which we could be tested, my medical school classmates and I soon divided ourselves into three groups. The first was the premed types— those still stuck in the premed mentality who were driven by competitiveness and the need to beat out their fellow students at all costs. The thirty or so members of this group made sure to attend each and every lecture and laboratory session; they sat in the first three rows of the large lecture hall and spent their time writing down, word for word, everything the lecturer said. They were certain that something was going to be said in the lecture which wasn't covered in the syllabus, some small bit of information which, sooner or later, would wind up in an examination question, and they would get the question right while everyone else got it wrong. Of course this scenario was never played out, but these students simply couldn't change their thinking.

The second group, the portion of the class to which I belonged, was made up of about a hundred students whose main motivation was guilt. Our logic went something like this: we knew we didn't have to attend lectures; we understood that everything we needed to know was included in the lecture notes, and that if we just spent our time at home studying we'd do fine. But we felt lax not coming to class; we felt it was our duty to appear every day and take up a seat. And so, every morning, all one hundred of us entered the lecture hall, took our regular seats toward the back of the room, and as the lecturer lowered the lights and began to show his slides we'd each, very quietly, open the copy of the *New York*

Times we'd brought with us to the crossword puzzle page; we'd fold the paper back and spend the next two hours finishing the puzzle. During those two preclinical years I became quite expert at doing the *Time*'s crosswords.

The third group was composed of the remaining fifty or so students who made up our class, who had enough strength of character to transcend the guilt of not showing up. These students would appear only periodically: they'd come on the first day of each course, the day the syllabus was distributed, and they'd return again the day the final was given. The rest of the time they were almost never seen within the confines of the Schweitzer campus.

My friend, Phil Marks, was a member of this group. Amazingly, Phil, one of the most intelligent people I've ever met, held a full-time job as a computer programmer in Cambridge, Massachusetts, during our first two years of medical school. Phil shared an apartment in the Bronx with another of our classmates but lived most of the time in an apartment in Cambridge. Phil would return to the Bronx the evening before each scheduled test. He would eat dinner with his roommate, then read through the course syllabus once or twice. Using this technique, Phil passed every single exam. Of course, he had to give up his job in his third year, when it was necessary to actually show up on the ward every day. But for the first two years, Phil earned enough money to pay his tuition, his rent, and his transportation; he even had enough to put a little away in savings.

As the lecturers droned on and on during those first two years, it didn't take long for the enthusiasm I'd felt at the start of medical school to diminish. Through hard work and long hours of studying, I somehow managed to pass all the first-year classes. But when the second year rolled around I became more discouraged, and keeping my nose to the grindstone was increasingly difficult. In October of that year I failed my first exam, in microbiology, and was forced to take a retest, which, luckily, I passed. By December, even after all I'd been through, I wasn't sure anymore that this was what I really wanted to do.

Just when things seemed to be at their worst we began a course called Physical Diagnosis, in which we learned how to take histories from and examine real patients. The beginning of P.D. heralded a change; we were finally moving from the preclinical into the clinical sciences. At last it appeared that I'd start learning the things I had come to medical school to learn. I spent a lot of time in P.D. and enjoyed the work immensely.

The entire third year of medical school is spent in clinical clerkships, rotations of varying lengths in each of the major specialties of modern medicine. Clinical clerks spend their time on the wards of hospitals, working closely with the interns and residents who provide most of the patient care. I started the clerkship year doing pediatrics, then moved to the general surgery service; after surgery I did psychiatry, internal medicine, and radiology, ending the year in obstetrics and gynecology. I enjoyed each of my clerkships. More important, the experience confirmed in my mind that I'd made the right decision; within a month of the start of my third year of school, I remembered what it was about medicine that had attracted me to the field in the first place.

2

It's 3 A.M.: Do You Know What Your Doctor Is Thinking?

Third-year clerkship in internal medicine, December 1976

"Can you give me a hand? Schwab just spiked a fever and I have to do a sepsis workup."

The intern's words couldn't have come at a worse time. It was a little after two-thirty in the morning, and after a day that had started more than nineteen hours before, my brain was about fried. As a student doing my clinical clerkship in internal medicine, I wasn't expected to spend the entire night in the hospital. On days when Al Barrister, the intern with whom I had been assigned to work at the start of the rotation, was scheduled to be on call, I was supposed to leave around midnight. In fact, just as Al poked his head into the house-staff lounge to ask for my help I was getting ready to leave, shoving my stethoscope, otoscope, and ophthalmosocope into my backpack, thinking about how wonderful it would be to get home and into my nice, warm bed. But it was now December, and the one thing I had learned in the months since I'd begun my first clinical clerkships in August, was that clerks must never, ever refuse when interns request help. So I nodded, left my backpack half packed, and sleepily followed Al down the hall toward the room near the end of 4 South which housed Mrs. Schwab's bed.

Mrs. Schwab was one of the first patients I had been assigned by the resident to follow during this clerkship, my fourth rotation. She was a tiny woman, eighty-six years old, who had been in excellent health until about a year before, when she'd awakened one morning with shortness of breath and swelling of her hands and feet. She hadn't thought much of these symptoms then, but when her breathing grew more labored later in the day she paid a visit to her regular doctor's office. That visit resulted in the first of what would become a series of emergency admissions to Jonas Bronck Hospital. During her initial admission, an X ray of Mrs. Schwab's chest revealed that the woman's heart was enlarged and that her lungs were filled with fluid; because of these and some other abnormalities, a diagnosis of congestive heart failure was made.

Congestive heart failure occurs when the heart, usually an extraordinarily efficient pump, begins to weaken. Because it is no longer able to propel the great quantities of oxygenated blood it receives from the lungs to the rest of the body, fluid backs up into the lungs. When these organs become choked, breathing is difficult and uncomfortable, and it is nearly impossible for the lungs to perform their task of removing carbon dioxide, a waste product of normal metabolism, from the blood and exchanging it for life-giving oxygen. Eventually, if untreated, patients with congestive heart failure die of respiratory insufficiency, essentially drowning in their own secretions.

Mrs. Schwab's heart failure hadn't gotten nearly to that point. On admission to Jonas Bronck that first time she had immediately been given supplemental oxygen to ease the burden on her lungs and had been started on both digoxin, a medication that improves the pumping power of the heart, making its contracting force more efficient, and Lasix, a potent diuretic that effectively removes all excess fluid from the lungs. Within the course of a few days Mrs. Schwab was restored to her old, healthy self. A limited workup was performed during her hospitalization to try to uncover some treatable cause for her heart's sudden breakdown, but nothing obvious was found. Mrs. Schwab's cardiac failure, it was concluded, had been a consequence of the normal aging process, a sign that her life was beginning to wind down.

Now stable on her new medications, she was discharged home to her apartment, where she did reasonably well for a few weeks. Although the drugs didn't completely agree with her, making her tired and somewhat listless, she was more or less able to pick up her life and carry on as usual, at least for a while. But then, one morning about a month after she was discharged from the hospital, she awoke with a new set of symptoms: this time she was nauseated and, during the course of the next three hours, vomited a half dozen times; she had no appetite for breakfast and was lethargic. Again, Mrs. Schwab wasn't initially overly concerned about these symptoms; she figured she was just coming down with the flu or some other winter virus. But because of her recently diagnosed heart condition she decided to check with her physician. He suggested that she come to his office right away, and her visit led to her second emergency admission to Jonas Bronck Hospital.

This time she was found to be in chronic renal failure. Like her heart, her kidneys seemed to be coming to the end of the road; for no good reason other than age, these organs had significantly deteriorated, no longer able effectively to remove from her blood the natural by-products of human metabolism such as lactic acid, potassium, and nitrogen. These and other chemicals normally eliminated by the kidneys had gradually built up to toxic levels in Mrs. Schwab's blood, finally causing the symptoms she first experienced that morning. If her renal failure had gone untreated, Mrs. Schwab would have died.

An emergency hemodialysis treatment was performed during her first day in the hospital. Her blood now cleansed, Mrs. Schwab's symptoms immediately improved. That second hospitalization lasted two full weeks, during which time she was put on a strict diet severely limiting the amount of salt and protein she was allowed to take in. Once on the diet Mrs. Schwab found that she felt better, and she was again discharged.

But for a second time her improvement proved to be short-lived. Within weeks, another episode of congestive heart failure occurred, requiring yet another admission to Jonas Bronck. After stabilization, her dosages of digoxin and Lasix were readjusted. But although the fine-tuning of her medications effectively got her cardiac problem under control, it further disturbed her renal function. Less than a month after her third discharge from the hospital she was back again, this time with acute kidney failure.

Mrs. Schwab's medical problems continued unmercifully throughout the year. The failure of her heart muscle and of her kidney function were only the beginning of the elderly woman's troubles. Since those first admissions she'd suffered two bouts of pneumonia, both of which landed her in the intensive care unit, hooked up by tubes to a mechanical ventilator; she'd had a minor stroke that left her right side slightly weaker than her left; and she'd developed hepatitis—a mild case that she contracted from one of the blood transfusions she had received to correct the chronic anemia stemming from renal insufficiency. But through all her ordeals—the ambulance rides, the middle-of-the-night visits to the emergency room, the hospitalizations, and the increasing complications of her treatment plan, Mrs. Schwab remained alert and sharp as a tack; she even managed to keep her sense of humor.

I was familiar with her medical history because Mrs. Schwab and I had spent a lot of time together during the days since her admission. This time it was because of her heart that she had been given a bed on 4 South, the internal medicine floor to which Al Barrister and I were assigned. On the Sunday before her admission, at the wedding of her great-niece on Long Island, Mrs. Schwab had strayed from her highly restrictive diet, cheating by eating a huge quantity of sour pickles. "I can't resist them," she told me between labored breaths through her oxygen mask when I came to take her history. "They're my biggest weakness." She had expended her allotment of sodium for entire weeks to come on those pickles and as a result had blown up like a balloon, retaining enough water to plunge her fragilely balanced system over the edge and into congestive failure. She had been admitted on Tuesday, two days after the wedding and one day after I started my rotation.

I liked Mrs. Schwab right away. Even though she was so sick that breathing was difficult, she was funny and outspoken, gently criticizing the emergency room staff for making her wait so long to be admitted and talking back to the ward nurses who, over the course of the previous year, had come to know her well. Speaking in her thickly accented English, she reminded me of the grandmother of my fiancée, Beth. Like Frieda, a spunky ninety-year-old who had come to America with her family at the age of sixteen to escape religious persecution in Russia, Mrs. Schwab had also immigrated as a teenager, from the same region in which Frieda had lived, for the same reason. And later, when we'd brought her cardiac failure somewhat under control and she was breathing easier and no longer required extra oxygen, Mrs. Schwab told me that I reminded her of one of her grandsons whom she'd encouraged to go to medical school, but who hadn't listened to her, choosing instead to become a rock musician. "He travels around with some cockamamie rock band," she told me. "What kind of a life is that for a nice Jewish boy?"

Managing Mrs. Schwab's congestive heart failure turned out to be easy. She responded well to the large dose of Lasix Al gave her through the intravenous line he had placed in her right hand as soon as she came up to 4 South from the emergency room: within an hour she began to mobilize the excess fluid she'd stored away, producing liters of urine. Within twelve hours she was breathing fairly comfortably. As she improved I found myself spending more time in her room, talking to her, rooting for her, hoping that this hospital stay would be a short one.

At first it looked as though her stay would indeed be short. On Wednesday morning, the day after she was admitted, Mrs. Schwab was doing so well that, during rounds, Al Barrister, in consultation with the team's senior resident and the attending physician, a cardiologist, decided that if she continued to improve at the rate she had up till then she could be discharged later in the day. But just as rounds were ending, before Al could begin to make any of the arrangements necessary for the patient's discharge—before anyone had even had a chance to let her know the good news—one of the nurses came to tell us that Mrs. Schwab had developed a fever. Al again reviewed the case with our senior resident, and the two of them decided to stand by and watch for a while, taking no immediate action, in hopes that the fever was a fluke, caused by nothing serious. If her temperature came down to normal by the next time it was taken, the resident agreed that we could still send Mrs. Schwab back home sometime later that day.

But it didn't come down to normal. When it was next checked at noon the thermometer read 102 degrees, dashing any chance that Mrs. Schwab would get an early discharge. Even worse, when Al and I examined her, trying to identify the source of her fever, we found that her breathing was again labored, and that rales—crackling sounds similar to the noise made when a piece of paper is crumpled—could be heard in the region of her chest which overlay the lower lobe of her left lung. Knowing that rales were indicative of a pulmonary infiltrate and that they hadn't been heard even when her congestive heart failure had been at its worst, Al concluded that Mrs. Schwab had probably developed pneumonia. Glumly, I helped him perform a complete sepsis workup. We drew blood from her tiny, easily collapsible veins for a complete blood count and for bacterial cultures, then obtained a sterile specimen of urine, also for culture.

Finally, after strapping a portable oxygen tank to her stretcher and placing an oxygen mask over the patient's face, I wheeled Mrs. Schwab down to the X-ray department to get a film of her chest. I tried during the trip to encourage her, telling her that everything was going to turn out fine. She didn't believe me, though; she was in too much respiratory distress.

Mrs. Schwab was right. At the time I took her down to the X-ray department her condition was far from fine: the X-ray confirmed the presence of a whopping pneumonia in the lower lobe of her left lung, which began a series of complications and setbacks that, over the next few days, left her close to death.

We began treating the pneumonia with ampicillin, one of the most commonly used antibiotics, but the fever persisted despite treatment. Then on Friday, forty-eight hours after the pneumonia had first been diagnosed, Mrs. Schwab suffered another dramatic setback: she developed hives all over her body as well as swelling of her face and tongue, a complication that compromised her breathing even more. Al concluded that these symptoms had been caused by anaphylaxis, an allergic reaction to the antibiotic, and quickly gave her a shot of epinephrine to reverse the swelling and respiratory problems. But even after he switched her to another antibiotic Mrs. Schwab's symptoms did not improve, and within hours she was sick enough to require transfer to the intensive care unit, where she was intubated and placed on a ventilator.

Worsening kidney failure followed. Mrs. Schwab's renal function, which had been marginal to begin with, simply collapsed, and by the weekend another emergency hemodialysis treatment was required. By Sunday afternoon her condition had deteriorated to such an extent that an informal conference was convened among the ICU staff. Mrs. Schwab, now on a ventilator, with a case of pneumonia that resisted the treatments we had offered, in worsening renal failure, and with a cardiac status that was shaky at best, seemed to be on an acutely downhill course. Considering the patient's age and her litany of medical problems, the staff decided that there was nothing more that could or should be done to prolong her life; it was suggested that her family be summoned so that, with their permission, plans could be made to cease all heroic medical intervention.

Mrs. Schwab's immediate family consisted of her three children, all of whom lived in the Los Angeles area, and her grandchildren, who were scattered throughout the United States. The ICU social worker, who had attended the conference, promptly set about trying to contact Mrs. Schwab's children. By Monday afternoon everyone had arrived—even the grandson who had been on the road with the cockamamie rock band. They swarmed in the family room of the ICU, each waiting for a turn to see the family's matriarch in her last illness. But when a nurse finally led them one by one to her bedside, the old woman didn't seem nearly as bad off as any of them had been led to believe.

Mrs. Schwab had rallied. Something inside her, some internal force, had made her fight on, had told her that the time was not yet right for her to die. On Sunday night her vital signs stabilized; by Monday morning she had regained enough of her old strength to begin to breathe on her own again, and as the day went on she required less and less assistance from the artificial ventilator. And while her grieving children and grandchildren stood at her bedside, we gladly began preparing to remove the breathing tube from her throat. No, no decision about withdrawing heroic care for Mrs. Schwab would be made on that day; almost miraculously, she had become her old self one more time. I silently cheered as, late that afternoon, the woman, now breathing spontaneously, sat up in her bed and, in a hoarse voice, asked, "So when can I go home already?"

She wasn't quite ready to go home just then, but by Tuesday morning she was well enough to be transferred out of the ICU and back to the general medicine floor. She appeared to be back to her baseline again. On rounds on Tuesday morning we repeated our discussion about discharge plans, deciding that she would be allowed to go home as soon as she'd completed the ten-day course of antibiotics which would ensure that her pneumonia was eradicated. And she continued to do well until late Thursday night, or, more correctly, early Friday morning, when, as I was packing up to leave for home, she once again became short of breath and developed a fever. As Al and I trudged down the hall toward her hospital room, stopping first in the ward's treatment room to pick up the supplies we needed for the sepsis workup, we both understood how serious the situation might be. But the two of us responded very differently to that understanding.

"I hate this!" Al said angrily as we walked down the hall.

I agreed, but didn't say anything more. Once in her room we found Mrs. Schwab looking much grayer and significantly less spunky than she'd been on the day I first met her, sitting straight up in bed, leaning forward, trying to catch her breath. Although she was in mild respiratory distress she could still speak without difficulty. "Is anything hurting you?" the intern asked, sounding angry.

"No," the patient answered.

"You have a fever again," Al continued, almost as if he were blaming her for the temperature spike. "We'll have to do some tests to find out what's causing it."

"More tests?" Mrs. Schwab asked. "More needles?"

"We have no choice," Al replied. And with that, we went to work.

While I washed Mrs. Schwab's left elbow with a gauze pad soaked in Betadyne, an antiseptic solution, Al set up the empty tubes and the bottles of culture broth into which we would squirt specimens of blood. As he bound a tourniquet tight around her upper arm I held Mrs. Schwab's hand in mine, trying to steady her arm so it wouldn't jerk when the needle entered through the skin.

Mrs. Schwab's veins were fragile, the result of a com-

bination of factors including her age, her horrendous year
of infirmity, and the numerous needle sticks she'd endured during the past week. To make matters worse, Al
didn't exactly have a light touch. He stuck the needle
under the skin of the patient's elbow, advanced it forward
as she cried out in pain, and . . . nothing happened.
"Damn!" he yelled over the woman's shouting as he
pulled the needle out of her arm.

"Did you get it?" Mrs. Schwab asked, feeling the
needle exit her skin. "Did you get what you needed?"

Al remained silent, so I answered the question: "No,
Mrs. Schwab; unfortunately, we'll have to try again."

The intern and I got set up a second time, preparing
to attempt to draw blood now from her right arm. I
scrubbed her elbow with Betadyne while Al prepared the
needle and syringe. Again she shouted as the needle entered her skin, and again the intern yelled "Damn!"
when no blood appeared in the needle's tubing. Pulling
the needle out, Al straightened up and, without uttering
a sound, stormed angrily out of the room.

After apologizing to Mrs. Schwab, telling her that we
hadn't gotten the blood and that we'd have to stick her a
third time, I rushed out after him. I saw him entering the
treatment room down the hall, where I found him angrily
pulling supplies from the shelves, needles and syringes
he'd need to try again to get the necessary blood specimens. "What's wrong?" I asked.

"I hate this," Al muttered. "I just hate it. Look at
what's happening here. Look at what I'm doing: it's three
o'clock in the morning; I have a full day tomorrow; I
have all these sick patients to get squared away in the
morning, and then I have clinic all afternoon. There's no
way I'll get out of this hospital before eight o'clock tomorrow night. I should be asleep now; that's the only
way I'll be any good for anything tomorrow. I should be
sleeping, but what the hell am I doing? I'm trying to get
blood out of the arm of a woman who should be dead.
I'm supposed to be doing a fucking sepsis workup on
somebody who's got no prognosis, no chance of surviv-

ing for more than a few days or a few weeks or at best
maybe another month or two, somebody who we'd be
leaving alone now if her fucking family hadn't come all
the way from California to tell us we had to do everything
possible to keep her alive. None of this makes any sense,
does it?''

"What do you mean, she should be dead?" I asked. I
was startled by Al's outburst, but I especially focused on
this one point. ·

"Just what I said: she should be dead. This woman
has multisystem failure. Her heart, her lungs, her kidneys, even her liver are all shot to hell. There's no way
anybody can do anything to fix her; all we'll ever be able
to do is palliate her, take care of the problem she has at
the moment so that it might temporarily go away. Then
we'll send her home and within another couple of days
she'll be back with something else. It's only a matter of
time—she's going to die soon; there's no doubt about it.
If she'd had the decency to die last weekend like she
should have I'd be in bed now, sound asleep; instead she
lived, so I've got to keep trying to get blood out of her
for this stupid sepsis workup.''

"I don't understand how you can talk like that," I
replied. "This is a person; she's got a mind; she's got
children and grandchildren who love her. She's not some
monster who's been sent here to keep you up at night.
How can you be so cruel?''

Al glared at me and shook his head. "You don't understand, do you?'' he said. "You just don't understand.'' Having collected all the supplies he needed, the
intern turned and walked out of the treatment room. I
followed him down the hall, back to Mrs. Schwab's bedside. Silently now, we attempted a third time to get blood
from the patient. Finding a small but sturdy vein in the
woman's right hand, Al was finally successful in getting
the quantity he needed.

Mrs. Schwab's fever turned out to be inconsequential;
no source was ever identified, and by the time her tem-

perature was taken again at four o'clock it had returned to normal. The rest of her hospital stay was unremarkable, and Mrs. Schwab was discharged home after completing the ten-day course of antibiotics for her pneumonia. She was not readmitted to Jonas Bronck Hospital again during the remainder of my eleven-week rotation in internal medicine, and I haven't seen or heard of her since the day she left 4 South.

I spent the rest of that December working closely with Al Barrister, and although we had no further confrontations, I didn't forget the words he said to me. It amazed me that someone who had already sweated and slaved his way through four years of medical school, who had completed six months of an internship in internal medicine, could be as heartless, as cold, and as self-centered as the angry, overtired intern I faced in the treatment room that early morning. I couldn't get over the fact that he cared more about his own welfare, about his own sleeping habits, than he did about the well-being of his patients. Someone like that, I thought at the time, shouldn't be allowed to work as a physician. Over the next few days I even considered reporting Al's behavior to the head of the internal medicine residency program in an attempt to get the guy thrown out, or at least to make sure he got some counseling. But after discussing the incident with a few of my classmates, I realized that turning him in would not only do Al little or no good, it would jeopardize my standing with the higher-ups in the department, which any medical student tries to avoid at all costs.

On my way home from the hospital that night I made a promise to myself: I swore that I would never allow myself to think about a patient the way Al Barrister thought about Mrs. Schwab. It was a promise that, I'm sorry to say, I have not been able to keep. Looking back on the episode now, I realize that I was unduly harsh on Al. The frightening truth is that it wasn't his fault. At some point during training, nearly every doctor has similar thoughts about one or more patients. This phenomenon is a product of night after night of going without sleep, the months and months of chronic exhaustion, the sadness and frustration and depression that compose the life of an intern. After some of the more nightmarish days and terror-filled nights that make up medical training, we all, sooner or later, wind up inhabited by the monster that awoke in the body of Al Barrister that early morning in the treatment room on 4 South.

But for the most part I enjoyed my third year of medical school. It was during that year that Beth and I were married. We had met as freshmen in college and dated ever since, but our courtship became complicated following graduation: we'd spent two of those years—the time I was in Ireland and my first year at Schweitzer, during which Beth worked as a technician in a microbiology lab in Boston—separated by hundreds of miles. Beth decided to come to New York at the beginning of my second year of medical school, enrolling as a graduate student in molecular biology at Columbia University. Since we were both concentrating on academic endeavors, finally getting married the next year allowed us to stabilize our social lives. We moved into a two-bedroom apartment in a building on the Schweitzer campus and became part of the school's small but tight-knit community of married couples.

I learned a great deal in all six of the clinical clerkships that composed that third year. Each one offered something different. In pediatrics, I enjoyed the contact with children and their families. I was touched by the fact that, no matter how sick they seemed when first entering the hospital, most children recovered quickly, leaving the ward after a few days nearly as good as new. While on surgery rotation I came to appreciate the hours of pure, intense concentration surgeons put in in the operating room, time during which they blot out all the mundane interruptions that characterize hospital life—the blaring of beepers and the piles of tedious scut work (jobs such as checking lab results, drawing blood, starting IVs, and so on)—in order to focus all their attention and skill on a single small square of skin and the diseased tissue underlying it. In internal medicine and radiology I was attracted to the intellectual challenge, the medical chess game engaged in by the doctors when a patient with an interesting or confusing set of symptoms appeared on the wards. In psychiatry I was awed by the complexity of disease that occurred in the patients I followed, the fascinating but often frightening spectrum of aberrations that can affect the human mind. And in obstetrics the joy accompanying the birth of a healthy infant drew me in.

The environment in which we clinical clerks worked was ideal for learning. As third-year students who still knew little about medicine, we were not directly responsible for patient care.

We were expected to be on the ward every third night, when the intern to whom we had been assigned was scheduled to be on call; we had to help with the scut work; and we did a certain number of write-ups—histories and physicals performed on new patients which were evaluated by the attending physicians—during the course of each rotation. But there was little pressure on us, and as a result that third year seemed to fly by. And then the fourth year began.

Although set in the same hospitals and occurring on the same wards as the third-year rotations, the fourth year of medical school brings a marked change in the level of performance required of medical students. During the five months of mandatory rotations in ambulatory medicine, in neurology, and in something called a subinternship (during which the student spends two months working as an intern), the student for the first time has direct responsibility for patients. And even though interns, residents, and attending physicians provide substantial back-up support, it is the student who first meets the patient in the emergency room; it is the student who takes the history, performs the physical exam, and develops a list of diagnostic possibilities; and it is the student who plans the workup to prove the diagnosis and then institutes a course of management to treat the prob-

lem. Naturally, with this increase in responsibility during
these five months of the fourth year of medical school
comes a significant amount of stress.

I began my fourth year at Schweitzer doing the mandatory rotation in ambulatory medicine; during July and
August of 1977, I worked in the emergency rooms and
clinics of Jonas Bronck Hospital. That July was spent in
adult medicine; in August, I worked on the pediatric side.

3

Life and Death 101

**Fourth-year ambulatory medicine rotation,
July–August 1977**

Hearing the commotion in the hallway outside the examination booth, I looked up from the tiny square of bed sheet on which I'd been concentrating for what seemed like days and gazed toward the door. It sounded as if a riot had broken out in the corridor: loud voices shouted over a rumbling noise, a sound like that made by a plane as it taxis for a takeoff. "I think he actually fell asleep." The surgical resident whom I was assisting didn't take his eyes off the scalp wound he was suturing on a patient who'd been almost too much for the two of us to handle when he came in. "I think I can manage it from here. Why don't you go out there and see what's going on."

I had been dying to hear those words for the past two hours. I'd been lying on top of a stretcher, trying my best to keep motionless the middle-aged man on whom the surgeon was working, a guy who had managed to walk through a plate glass window earlier that afternoon. The patient, who had been exceedingly inebriated at the time of his accident, had a huge, deep gash across his forehead which was gushing blood when the cops had brought him into the emergency room, kicking and screaming, a little over two hours before. While the senior surgical resident tried to suture the wound the man fought, bit,

33

screamed, and cursed, and the surgeon, seeing that he would need help in order to get the wound repaired, requested that a large medical student be sent over to hold the patient down. That's when I first got involved. I had been lying on top of this drunk ever since, trying to keep him still, smelling his foul, alcoholic breath, taking his bites and punches and verbal abuse in stride. Now, after nearly two hours, my arm and neck muscles were aching and the rest of my body was fatigued, and when the surgeon finally suggested that I check out the commotion in the hallway I was off the patient and at the door of the examination booth almost instantaneously.

On the other side of the door was a stretcher being wheeled toward me at breakneck speed by Donna Richards, the head nurse of the emergency room. A paramedic ran alongside the gurney, pumping on an ambu bag, a rubber bladder that forces air into the lungs. On top of the gurney, straddling the abdomen of the apparently critically ill man, kneeled a second paramedic, this one performing cardiac massage.

After allowing the stretcher to pass I followed, running close behind. They were headed toward the emergency room's critical care area as fast as they could travel. Since I was one of the first to arrive on the scene I was ordered by Donna to replace the paramedic who'd been performing cardiac compressions. I took the man's place almost automatically, hopping up on the stretcher and beginning to press down on the patient's breastbone with the heel of my hand every few seconds, just as the paramedic had done. The transfer from paramedic to medical student took place without a single beat being missed. I was glad to take over the job: at last I was doing something, making a real contribution to the care of a patient. I knew that, at that moment, these chest compressions were keeping the man on the stretcher alive, and it felt good finally to be doing something helpful.

It was the beginning of July, the start of my fourth and final year of medical school, and I was beginning to think

I had wasted the last three years of my life. I had begun the mandatory two-month rotation in ambulatory medicine in the outpatient department at Jonas Bronck Hospital just a few days before. Although I entered the rotation, during which I would be working in the hospital's emergency rooms and clinics, with a full year of ward experience behind me, it had rapidly become clear that I actually knew very little about how to evaluate and care for new, undiagnosed patients. During my clerkships I'd shown that I was great at following orders given by interns, residents, and attending physicians with whom I was assigned to work; I had demonstrated that I could draw blood, write chart notes, and even start intravenous lines on most patients. But all of my work had been supervised. The very brief experience I'd had in the emergency room so far had already shown me that I didn't know the first thing about assessing and evaluating patients who came in for treatment. I seemed to be helpless when it came to putting facts together, synthesizing a differential diagnosis, and planning the workup and treatment of the patients I was supposed to be caring for. During my first few days in the emergency room I had done little other than stand around, watching closely as the real doctors went about their work. This routine quickly became tedious and disappointing, making me angry that I was so ill prepared by my three long years of medical school for the real job of being a doctor.

But finally, after four days, I was getting the chance to do something helpful. The patient on the stretcher was an elderly man who looked as if he'd been pretty badly beaten up. Looking down at him while repeatedly forcing the heels of my hands against the lower third of his breastbone, I saw that the right side of his head was a gory mess; his skull looked as if it had been bashed in, and there was a series of large gashes around the area, lacerations that were spilling thin rivulets of blood from his scalp with every downward thrust I administered to his chest. Dried, caked blood covered everything; it had already congealed in the man's gray hair, turning it into a sticky, matted mess; it had pooled in the hollows of his eyes and coated his ears and nose; it had soaked through the cervical collar the paramedics had placed around his neck when they picked him up.

The man must have been in cardiopulmonary arrest when the paramedics first reached him because he'd been intubated in the field; that is, the ambulance team had passed a plastic endotracheal tube into the man's mouth and forced it down through his vocal cords until it came to rest in his trachea in order to provide artificial ventilation during the time it took to get him to the hospital. Now blood had even begun to clot over the adhesive tape used to hold the endotracheal tube in place. I suspected that the man had been mugged by one of the many low-lifes who had begun populating the Bronx in alarming numbers over the last few years; it looked as though, in an attempt to get his wallet, the poor guy had been hit over the head with a baseball bat or some other blunt, heavy object. I knew from my third-year clerkships that such was the usual scenario when an elderly person in this condition was admitted to Jonas Bronck Hospital.

But when the hospital's trauma team arrived at the critical care area, I learned the real story. The team, headed by Trevor Jones, the hospital's chief surgeon, and composed of two general surgeons and an anesthesiologist, had been stat paged over the loudspeaker system as soon as the man came through the door. The team members appeared on the run less than three minutes after the stretcher came to rest. "We picked him up at the corner of Fordham Road and the Grand Concourse," reported the paramedic—the one who just minutes before had been performing chest compressions—while Dr. Jones briefly went about examining the patient. "A hit and run. He was in complete arrest when we arrived on the scene: there was no heart rate and no spontaneous respirations. We intubated, started a line"—he pointed to the large-bore needle that had been stuck into the patient's right arm through which an intravenous solution known as lactated Ringers was dripping—"and initiated CPR. He hasn't breathed on his own since we picked him up."

"How about his heart?" the chief surgeon asked. "Has there been any spontaneous rhythm?"

"It's been flatline all the way in," the second paramedic answered.

"There's been no response at all to pain," the first paramedic continued. Even I knew this was a sign that the patient was in a deep coma. "But his pupils have been equal and reactive."

That fact, evidence that the man's brain stem, the portion of the central nervous system which controls such vital activities as heart rate, respirations, and reflexes, was still performing some of its functions, was good news: the man had some chance of surviving the trauma. I pumped even harder and faster on the man's chest.

But Trevor Jones wasn't impressed by the paramedic's statement. The chief surgeon, a short man with a bushy brown beard who, as head of the trauma team, spent so much time at this end of the emergency room that it sometimes seemed as if he lived here, said, "Well, they might have been equal and reactive in the wagon, but they sure as hell aren't now." Dr. Jones had been shining a flashlight into the old man's eyes. "They're both fixed and dilated. He must have just herniated. Get neurosurgery down here, stat!"

Over the course of the next half hour, while the thrusts of my hands continued to pump the patient's blood through his heart and to his body, the members of the trauma team, aided by the neurosurgery resident on call that day, did everything they could to keep the man going. They gave him medications to try to get his heart beating again on its own; using a power drill, they carved a burr hole through his skull to relieve the dangerous increase in pressure from the swelling in his brain; with the electricity of a cardioverter, they tried to shock the man's heart back into action. But nothing worked. After everything failed, when it became clear to all of us assembled in the critical care area that the man had had it, that the injuries to his head had done too much permanent damage to his central nervous system, the chief surgeon finally brought events to a close. "He's dead," Dr. Jones said matter-of-factly. "Let's declare him. That's it; thank you all."

I reluctantly stopped pumping, and the members of the trauma team, the neurosurgeon, and the nurses who had assisted in the resuscitation slowly began to drift away from the critical care area. I stood there, staring down at the lifeless body that, mainly through the actions of my hands, had just seconds before been alive. I had an odd sensation in my gut, a feeling I didn't understand at that moment. Sure, I was upset, disappointed that this man, the first patient to whose care I had substantially contributed during my time in the emergency room, had died. But it was something more than that, some feeling I couldn't quite explain. I went to the sink to wash up; during the course of my pumping on his chest, my hands had become sticky and stained reddish brown with the man's blood. As I scrubbed I thought about what it was that was bothering me, that was making me feel so uneasy.

It was then that I remembered my grandfather.

The call had come late on a Friday evening in November. I'd been lying in bed, almost asleep, when I heard the phone ring. My mother answered it in my parents' bedroom down the hall. Though I couldn't hear anything that was said on the phone, I could tell the conversation was short, lasting only about a minute, and I clearly heard my mother's scream, my brain leaping from its groggy state to full consciousness as she started to cry. Determined to find out what was happening, I jumped out of bed and began running, but was intercepted in the hallway by my father, who had been coming to get me. "Your grandfather just passed away," he told me. "He was hit by a car." Consumed with emotion, he said nothing more.

My grandfather had been returning home from Friday

night services at the synagogue to which he'd belonged since settling in the Bronx more than thirty years before. He had been attempting to cross the Grand Concourse, just south of Fordham Road, just as he'd done hundreds of times before. But this time was different: a car approached from the north, well over the speed limit; barreling down the Concourse, running red light after red light, it struck my grandfather as squarely as if the driver had been aiming for him, dragging his body nearly two hundred feet following the impact. The driver must have been aware of what had happened; he had to have known that he'd hit a pedestrian, and that there was a good chance the man he'd hit had been killed instantly. But the witnesses at the scene, my grandfather's friends and longtime fellow congregants at the synagogue, swore that not only had the driver not stopped his car, he'd barely even slowed down. Almost immediately, they told the police, the car had been gone, continuing its speeding southbound journey down the Concourse.

One of the bystanders had called an ambulance, and my grandfather was rushed to Jonas Bronck Hospital— brought to this very emergency room, settled into this same critical care area. He was probably worked on by a trauma team led by one of Trevor Jones's predecessors; perhaps a fourth-year student at the Schweitzer School of Medicine, just beginning his outpatient rotation in the adult emergency room and frustrated because of his lack of experience and expertise, performed cardiac compressions, thrusting the heels of his hands against my grandfather's breastbone, happy for the chance to be doing something, anything, that might help a patient. And in the end, I guess, the chief surgeon—realizing that the patient's injuries were too severe, that that anonymous, speeding hit-and-run car had wreaked too much damage, that no physician, however skilled or talented, could undo what had been done in the instant of impact— declared my grandfather dead, sending the members of the trauma team slowly drifting away from the critical care area, sending my parents and the rest of my family into mourning, and taking away the only grandparent I'd ever known.

Standing over the sink in the trauma area, I scrubbed my hands steadily for a good five minutes. They weren't all that dirty or stained; the dried blood had come clean during the first rinsing. But still I stood there, rubbing my hands over and over again under the cool running water. I needed time to compose myself, to stop the tears that were forming in my eyes. I didn't want to cry, not now, on what was only my fourth day in the emergency room. I'd learned during my clinical clerkships that doctors weren't supposed to cry when one of their patients died, that tears shed at such a time were interpreted as a sign of weakness. So I stood there, soaping and rinsing, again and again, until I finally had my emotions under control.

After drying my hands on a paper towel, I returned to the side of the gurney. Two New York City cops had arrived on the scene by now; one was writing in a pocket-sized spiral notebook while the other drank coffee from a Styrofoam cup. Meanwhile Donna Richards was searching through the dead man's wallet, looking for some form of identification. "It's a damn shame," I heard her say to the cops as she shook her head slowly from side to side. "It's getting to the point where you take your life into your hands every time you go out to the grocery store to get a carton of milk. I can't believe what's happening in this city."

"Having any luck?" I asked as she continued rummaging through the wallet.

"I've got his Social Security card," she answered, waving the ragged-edged, worn piece of paper in the air. "His name's Isaac Tepperman. He doesn't seem to have a driver's license or anything that has a phone number or address on it." She searched a little more, while slowly shaking her head. "A guy like this—he's got to have a wife, and kids, and grandchildren. I'll tell you one thing: I'm not exactly looking forward to telling them what happened. . . ."

I'd never known who had made the phone call to my mother that Friday night or exactly what words were said to her during the brief conversation. Until that moment it had never occurred to me to wonder. "Are you the one who has to tell them?" I asked.

She nodded. "That's part of the head nurse's job," she answered. "And it sure as hell isn't my favorite." Just then, from the deepest recesses of Isaac Tepperman's wallet, the nurse pulled out a carefully hand-printed identification card. "Bingo!" she said. "Here it is." Tossing the wallet back onto the stretcher, the nurse started toward the wall phone. "Well, wish me luck," she sighed. "Maybe nobody'll be home."

That's when the idea came into my head. In silence, I debated it very briefly: should I volunteer to take the task, entering an area into which I'd never before wandered? Or should I ignore the urge, take the easy way out, let Donna do it, and go back to watching the ER doctors do their jobs? Nothing I'd learned so far in medical school, no course work or ward experience, had even remotely prepared me for anything like talking to the family of a man who had suddenly and unexpectedly died. I didn't know how it was supposed to be handled, what was supposed to be said. My hands became cold and clammy as I made my decision. "Hold on a minute, Donna," I said, just as the nurse was picking up the phone. "Do you mind if I make the call?"

"Are you kidding?" the nurse asked. When I shook my head, she said, "Do you know what you're getting yourself into? This isn't exactly a party. Do you have any idea how to handle it?"

"No," I replied. "But I know how they're going to feel." And without another word, I took Isaac Tepperman's identification card from the nurse's hand and nervously began to dial the number.

Speaking to Isaac Tepperman's wife that afternoon was by far the most difficult task I performed during the month I spent in the adult emergency room. Hanging on the phone, listening as the woman shrieked the way my own mother had cried out years before, and then, later, standing by her, trying to comfort her as she grieved over her husband's body in the trauma area was the most involvement I was to have with any patient or family during my rotation. For much of the rest of my time in the adult emergency room I remained an observer, rarely getting the opportunity to do much on my own.

But my experience changed at the beginning of August, when I started working in the pediatric outpatient department. I'm not sure exactly what happened, whether it was the system that was different or that I'd simply found my confidence, but in the first few days of the month I had the chance to see patients in the pediatric emergency room on my own, and I accepted the challenge without hesitation. In the pediatric ER I was allowed to see any child who wasn't critically ill, form opinions about diagnoses, and make management plans based on those opinions, making sure to check before doing anything with the resident or attending physician in charge. I thus gained experience in evaluating sick children, and my faith in my clinical skills grew. In fact, by the end of the month I had come to feel so secure about my abilities that, when one of the chief residents approached me and asked if I'd mind covering the emergency room as "early bird" on the last morning of August, I eagerly accepted the challenge. What a mistake!

At that time it was the job of the early bird, a position usually filled by a junior or senior resident, to staff the emergency room single-handedly between the hours of six and nine on weekday mornings. The early bird relieved the night float, the house officer who worked alone in the ER from eleven to six. It was the early bird's responsibility to keep the place under control and to see all patients who registered for care between the time he or she arrived and the time the day crew reported for work. During the last week of that August the person who had been scheduled to work as early bird came down with chicken pox. Although the chief residents tried to get the schedule covered, one morning remained when no other house officer could be found to fill in, and in desperation they asked me to help out. And so, at a little before six o'clock on the morning of Wednesday, August 31, 1977, after a long, sleepless night mostly spent worrying, I left our apartment, headed for Jonas Bronck Hospital.

As I arrived in the emergency room that morning I found Mark Miller, the senior resident who'd been on duty as night float, sitting in an examination booth, busily scribbling some notes on a chart. "How was your night?" I asked, sitting down in the chair next to his.

"I swear," Mark answered, "if I live to be a hundred, I'll never understand why anybody would bring a kid to the emergency room at five o'clock in the morning for a diaper rash. Can you believe it? A fucking diaper rash! I mean, for Christ's sake, the kid wasn't even complaining about it!" He signed his name at the bottom of the chart and wearily continued: "Look, I'm supposed to be able to go home as soon as the early bird shows up, but since you're not really supposed to be working here unsupervised, the chief residents kind of asked me to hang around until nine."

"You mean you're staying?" I asked, relieved.

"I can't exactly leave you here alone," the resident said. "I mean, it's not even legal for you to be here by yourself. So I don't see where I've got a whole lot of choice."

After I thanked him profusely, Mark went on: "It's pretty quiet now—I've cleared out all the charts, and there's nobody waiting to be seen. So if it's all right with you, I'm going to go into the isolation room and try to take a nap."

"Sure," I answered, "as long as you don't mind being woken up if I have a problem."

"I expect you to wake me up if you have a problem," he responded, "but it doesn't make a whole lot of sense for me to hang around out here when there's nothing that needs to be done. You see Lynn over there?'' he asked, gesturing toward a nurse who was making a fresh pot of coffee in the nurses' station. ''She's the night nurse. She's great, and she knows more pediatrics than nine tenths of the house staff. If you have any problems, Lynn's the first person you should talk to. And if she can't help you, you know where to find me.'' With those words, Mark shuffled off to the back of the emergency room and into the room usually used to isolate children with infectious diseases.

After introducing myself to Lynn and trying to explain to her what a fourth-year medical student was doing working as early bird, I returned to the examination booth just vacated by Mark and, taking a seat, began to pray that I'd get lucky and that no patients would register to be seen before nine o'clock. But my prayers weren't granted: at a little past seven a screaming five-year-old and his mother showed up at the registration desk. ''He was bitten by our dog about an hour ago,'' I heard the woman, obviously annoyed at having to come to the emergency room so early in the morning, tell Lynn. After getting the boy, who was hysterical, and his mother into the examination booth, I tried to inspect the kid's left arm. Although he was shrieking at the top of his lungs, becoming almost dangerous when I got anywhere near him, I managed to see all I needed to see; he had a couple of scratches and one small puncture hole over the back of his hand. ''What kind of dog was it?'' I asked.

''A German shepherd,'' the mother replied, still sounding angry. ''She's big, but she's gentle as a lamb. She normally wouldn't hurt a fly, unless she's provoked. I don't know what he did to her, but it must have been something terrible.'' These words from his mother, and the glare that accompanied them, brought the boy's crying to a crescendo.

Not having a clue as to what needed to be done for this patient, I excused myself and began heading toward the isolation room. But Lynn intercepted me before I'd made it even halfway back there. "Where do you think you're headed, pal?" she asked.

"The isolation room," I answered meekly.

"You're planning to wake up the resident for a dog bite?" she asked.

"He told me to get him if I needed any help," I answered.

"Look, that boy's been working all night; he needs a rest. You need help with a dog bite, you ask me, okay? A kid with meningitis comes in, then we can wake up Mark. *Comprende?*"

Intimidated, I nodded and asked, "Well, what should I do?"

"First you check to see if his tetanus shots are up to date. If they're not, I'll be more than happy to lay one on him. Then you give him a seven-day supply of penicillin and tell him to stay as far away from that dog as he can get. What the hell's a kid doing getting bitten by a German shepherd at six in the morning, anyway?"

I didn't answer, but turned and walked back toward the boy, who had finally stopped screaming, and his mother, who'd heard the entire exchange between the night nurse and me, and I did exactly as Lynn had instructed. By seven-thirty they were on their way out of the emergency room; before departing, the mother made sure to stop to thank Lynn for all her help.

I was beginning to relax again when the paramedics arrived at a little after eight. There were two of them, one with brown hair and the other with red; they were dressed identically in forest green uniforms and they carried matching walkie-talkies strapped to their belts. "Morning, Lynn," the brown-haired guy said as they approached the nurses' station. "How's business?"

"Fine, until you two showed up," the nurse replied. "What little bundle of joy do you have for us this morning?"

"We've got a SIDS in the back of our wagon," the red-haired guy said. I got to my feet and started walking toward the nurses' station when I heard that. I knew SIDS stood for sudden infant death syndrome.

"A SIDS?" Lynn asked, rising hurriedly. "You think you might want to bring the kid in? You think we might want to do some resuscitation here?"

"No resuscitation's needed on this one," the brown-haired paramedic responded slowly, shaking his head. "The mother found the kid cold and stiff in her crib at a little after seven."

"Her pupils were fixed and dilated when we got there," the red-haired one added, "and the corneas were already clouded over. She's been dead for at least a couple of hours."

"We don't even want to bring her in," the brown-haired guy said. "All we need to do is have someone come out to the wagon and declare her, and we'll take her straight down to the morgue."

From my position near the nurses' station I silently began inching my way toward the isolation room, but Lynn caught sight of my movement out of the corner of her eye and shouted, "Come on over here, Bob."

"Don't you think Mark ought to take this one?" I pleaded, yet obeying the nurse's command and edging slowly back toward the group. "I don't even know what to do."

"There really isn't anything you have to do," Lynn said. "You just go out there, make sure there's no heart-beat, and say the kid's dead. It's no big deal."

"What about her parents?" I asked, panicked. "What do I say to them?"

"You don't have to worry about that," the brown-haired paramedic replied. "They didn't come with us; they had to get dressed. They'll find their way over here sometime later."

"We'll call the priest and have him talk with them when they get here," the nurse added. "Better get moving now, before a busload of patients shows up and we start getting backed up."

Complying with Lynn's orders, I followed the two

paramedics out through the adult emergency room and into the hospital's ambulance port. Walking along behind them, I thought about the task before me. And my skin began to crawl.

I had been involved with patients who'd died—had worked on some, including Isaac Tepperman, at the very moment of death—but someone else had always been around, a more senior person who could take charge and do what needed to be done, including declaring the patient dead. Now there was no one else; I was alone, and for the first time I was in charge.

She was lying on a stretcher, strapped to a side rail in the back of the ambulance. She was covered with a blanket, but I could clearly make out the bulge that was her head, the one that was her trunk, the ones that were her legs. Even though it was already nearly ninety degrees outside and must have been over a hundred in the rear compartment of the ambulance, goose bumps sprouted on my skin and a chill ran down my spine. My first impulse was to run, but when I turned and tried to leave the back part of the ambulance the paramedics were outside, waiting for me. "All you have to do is say the word and we'll cart her down to the morgue," the red-haired one said.

Unable to escape, I whispered, "She's . . . she's dead."

"You haven't even uncovered her yet, Doc," he said.

"You really can't declare her unless you've actually examined her," the brown-haired one added.

Reluctantly, I headed back into the rear of the ambulance and slowly lowered the blanket. First the child's light brown hair was visible; then her forehead and her eyes came into view; then her nose and mouth appeared; and finally, there was the whole face.

She was beautiful. With fine, doll-like features, she looked almost too perfect to be real. "She's four months old," one of the paramedics said from behind, his voice shattering the tense silence, causing me to jump slightly. "Her parents' first baby."

Looking at her, I suddenly didn't believe she was dead. I yanked the blanket down, exposing her chest, and pulled out my stethoscope. Listening hard, concentrating all my efforts on trying to hear heart sounds. I was sure there was something there. "She's got a rate," I said in a panic. "Her heart's beating about 120 times a minute."

"Bullshit," the red-haired paramedic said, entering the ambulance, tearing the stethoscope from my ears, and putting the earpieces into his. After listening in silence for a few seconds, he said, "There's nothing there, Doc. You must have been hearing your own heart."

He handed the stethoscope back to me. When I put the earpieces into my ears and pressed it again to the infant's chest I knew he was right: I had been hearing my own heart as it pounded away within my chest at nearly twice the normal rate. Listening now, I realized there was nothing coming from the baby girl. "She is dead," I finally sighed, and quickly the paramedics re-covered the body in the blanket and prepared to drive off.

It was then that the tears came. Almost two months after I'd kept myself from crying at the time of Isaac Tepperman's death, I found that I could hold them back no longer. So I stood, alone in the ambulance port, crying inconsolably on that hot August morning.

After a few minutes Lynn came out to find me. "Move it, pal. This isn't rest period." But then, coming closer and seeing the state I was in, she put her arm around my shoulder and gently led me back into the emergency room.

Inside, Mark was awake and busy seeing a patient. The ER seemed to have come alive during the fifteen short minutes I'd been outside. Lynn led me to the now empty isolation room and called Mark over, stat. The resident immediately left his patient, saying as he entered the room, "This better be important." After taking one look at me sitting in a chair, holding my head in my hands, and sobbing softly to myself, he asked, "What happened, Bob?"

When I couldn't answer, Lynn spoke. "I sent him out to declare a SIDS and I found him like this out in the ambulance port."

"Your first dead baby?" Mark asked. I nodded. "I remember mine," he said, flopping down on the other chair in the room. "A kid who fell out of a fifth-story window during the summer of my internship. It's funny; he barely had a scratch on him. He looked fine, except for the fact that he was stone dead. I felt horrible. I had nightmares about him for months. I'm sorry it had to happen to you."

I had calmed down a little by then. Mark and Lynn stayed with me as long as they could, but a little before nine they were called out for an emergency: a ten-year-old had been brought in by ambulance in the midst of a long convulsion. I remained in the isolation room for nearly two hours. At about ten-thirty, when I felt I could once again cope with life, I stepped out of the room into an ER buzzing with activity, and I went to put in the last few hours of my rotation in the outpatient department.

Nothing in the course of medical education today readies the future physician for dealing with the death of a patient. Medical schools do not offer any organized method of preparing for the inevitability of a patient's death; students can't learn about talking to the dying patient or his family from lectures or videotapes; no book tells would-be doctors what to say when coming face to face with the parents of a child who has just unexpectedly passed away; no syllabus teaches students how they should (or will) feel when a patient dies, or how to cope with feelings of inadequacy or helplessness when these events do occur. Such lessons must be learned through experience—both during the years of training and in student's pre-medical school lives. Doctors must rely on their intuition and their past experiences to guide them through these difficult times.

It was during my two-month rotation in the outpatient department that I confronted death alone for the first time. Many insights flashed through my mind during those brief episodes in the emergency rooms of Jonas Bronck Hospital. I thought of my grandfather's death, and of the deaths of other relatives and family friends that had taken place during my childhood. I began to have some awareness of my own mortality, of the reality that someday I would be like that old man lying on the gurney at the back of the trauma area. And I discovered that, for some patients, death is inevitable—that no matter how hard I tried, how much I did, or how much I cared, some of my patients simply would not survive.

Until that rotation I had been learning only about the role of the physician in sustaining life. During July and August of 1977 I learned a few things about the doctor's role at the time of death.

Half of the fourth-year curriculum at Schweitzer was composed of mandatory rotations. For the rest of the year we students were encouraged to immerse ourselves in elective courses, working in areas that particularly interested us or filling in some of the holes in our knowledge resulting from deficiencies in our previous experience. It was for the latter reason that I decided to spend November of my senior year taking an elective in infectious diseases.

4

The Zoology Lesson

**Fourth-year elective in infectious diseases,
November 1977**

Somewhere along the line I'd developed a bad case of
infectious disease phobia. It was the subspecialty of
medicine about which I knew least. My problem began
early in medical school: at the start of the second year I
failed the final exam in microbiology. Then during the
clinical clerkships of my third year my mind always
seemed to wander off during rounds whenever the attending physician or senior resident turned the discussion
to viruses, bacteria, or fungi. My lack of knowledge
about infectious diseases troubled me: in my future life
as an intern and resident, having a firm grasp of the diagnosis and treatment of communicable processes would
be of extreme importance. And so, I reluctantly signed
up for the infectious disease elective that was offered at
Jonas Bronck Hospital.

On Tuesday morning, November 1, 1977, the first day
of the course, the infectious disease team assembled as
it usually did, promptly at eight A.M., within the warm,
moist confines of the bacteriology lab on the sixth floor
of the hospital. After the team had made quick rounds
through the medical and surgical wards to check the temperature charts and vital sign sheets of all the patients on
whom it had been asked to offer advice over the previous

week, I was ordered to go see a new patient on 4 East, one of the internal medicine wards. Fred Stein, the senior resident in charge of the group that month, told me to do a complete history and physical exam on the patient. "You're going to have to present her to our attending during rounds this afternoon," he said before sending me off, "so make sure you know enough about the woman so you don't wind up making a complete fool of yourself."

Filled with the confidence the resident's remarks had instilled in me, I walked over to 4 East and quickly identified the chart of the patient on whom an infectious disease consultation had been requested. Mrs. Iqbal was not the typical Jonas Bronck Hospital patient with whom I had become familiar during my previous clinical experiences. A well-groomed, mentally intact middle-aged Indian woman, Mrs. Iqbal was neither an alcoholic, nor a drug abuser, nor demented. In reviewing her chart, I found that she had been admitted to the hospital five days before for evaluation of an unremitting fever that had been present for more than a month. The initial workup performed by the 4 East ward team during those first few days of Mrs. Iqbal's inpatient stay included a massive number of blood tests and cultures of just about every type of body fluid that could be sampled using a twenty-two-gauge spinal needle. By her fifth day in the hospital, every one of those tests had come back normal; Mrs. Iqbal's fever, however, persisted, her temperature spikes surpassing 101 degrees each day. With nothing positive to go on, the 4 East team was stumped and it had requested assistance from the infectious disease service; what it got, unfortunately for everyone involved, was me.

After finishing my review of her chart, I found Mrs. Iqbal in her room where I chatted with her for well over an hour. She was a nice woman who seemed bored and more than a little lonely in the isolation room in which she had been placed, so she didn't seem to mind talking to me, even though she understood from the outset that, as a fourth-year medical student, it was very unlikely I would be able to come up with anything that might help her. At the start of our time together she recounted for me the same story of her illness she'd told to everyone else who had previously inquired: she had been in excellent health, with no symptoms or signs of disease, until sometime around the end of September, when suddenly, without warning, the fever had first appeared. Initially she figured she'd just picked up a case of the flu that had been going around and hadn't given it much thought. But after two weeks had passed and in spite of the fact that she had stayed home in bed, drunk plenty of fluids, and taken two aspirin tablets religiously every four hours, the fever persisted, she began to get worried. She then paid a visit to the Jonas Bronck emergency room, but when nothing abnormal was found by the doctor who examined her, she was sent home again with instructions to return in a week or two if the fever continued. When another two weeks had passed and the fever just didn't seem to want to quit, she returned to the ER. It was then decided to admit her to the hospital for evaluation.

The intern's admission note in Mrs. Iqbal's chart paralleled what she said, but I didn't stop with just that basic story. Being a medical student and not knowing exactly which facts were important and which weren't, I asked that poor woman about everything I could think to ask. I went on and on, filling page after page of progress-note paper with seemingly worthless bits of information: I did a complete family history, a menstrual and pregnancy history, a social and travel history. And then a frightening thought occurred to me: in my attempt to uncover the key piece of information which might solve the puzzle of what was causing Mrs. Iqbal's fever, I suddenly realized that I must sound just like my classmate, the dread Phil Nirenstein, as he'd hammered away at Mr. Stevenson, a man who had been admitted to our ward the year before when we were doing our clerkships in internal medicine.

* * *

I hated Phil Nirenstein. He was the kind of guy who always tried to outdo and outshine everyone else, to make himself look good to the discredit of others. He was easily the most competitive person I had ever met, the ultimate premed personality—one of those who spent the first two years of medical school seated in the front rows of the lecture hall, scribbling down everything the lecturer said. Nirenstein never allowed the fact that he'd been accepted to medical school interfere with the way he conducted himself, and through his intense competitiveness and lack of compassion, he made life difficult for me. And ever since our first year of school, I'd wanted to kill the guy.

Back in July of 1976, at the beginning of our third year, the class had been subdivided into six groups of students who rotated together through each of the clinical clerkships. On the morning the assignments were expected to be posted, I remember praying to God that Nirenstein wouldn't end up in the same group as me. But alas, my prayers went unanswered; when the lists went up on the bulletin board, under the column headed GROUP C I found the name NIRENSTEIN, PHILIP listed directly below MARION, ROBERT. My heart sank as I grasped that indeed, as I proceeded through my clinical clerkship rotations for the next year, Nirenstein and I would be permanently linked.

The first few rotations hadn't gone badly. Nirenstein, though still absurdly competitive, managed to keep himself reasonably under control. But then our rotation in internal medicine began, and Nirenstein reverted to form.

Since our first days in medical school Nirenstein had never made his desire to go into internal medicine a secret. By the time we started the rotation the guy pretty much had his whole life mapped out: he would graduate from Schweitzer with honors, do his internship and residency at the Massachusetts General Hospital in Boston, and go on to an equally prestigious fellowship program in cardiology. He would then establish himself in a high-volume private practice and wind up making millions. The fulfillment of his dream rested heavily on his being offered a place at Mass. General, and in order to accomplish this goal he would have to get a grade of honors in this clerkship (although the preclinical courses had been graded on a pass/fail basis, grades for the clerkships included honors, reserved for the top 10 percent of all students.) And so, once again letting his pent-up exuberance run wild, Nirenstein nearly knocked himself out trying to impress the attending physicians, the senior doctor and the faculty member responsible for running the ward—that is, those ultimately evaluating our performance.

During December 1976, the first month of the rotation, Nirenstein's plan had worked to perfection. The attending physician that month happened to be a cardiologist. One Monday morning early in the month, Nirenstein showed up at our daily teaching rounds clutching a textbook entitled *The Sick Sinus Syndrome*. He and the intern with whom he was working had admitted a patient with this unusual condition when they were on call the previous Saturday, and Nirenstein had spent the entire previous day—his only day off for the past two weeks—in the library reading about it. None of the rest of the students in the group even had a clue as to what the hell sick sinus syndrome was; I figured it must have something to do with the air-filled structures in the face that get clogged when one comes down with a head cold, but it turned out that I wasn't even close: sick sinus syndrome refers to a dysfunction in the conduction system of the heart, the cells that control the cardiac rhythm.

Although none of the rest of us knew anything about the disorder, Nirenstein certainly did—through his reading he had learned everything there was to know about sick sinuses, and he and our attending physician spent all of rounds that day in a discussion that was so technical and sophisticated that afterward even our team's senior resident admitted that he hadn't been able to follow what they said. The attending physician was clearly very impressed with young Nirenstein. For the rest of the month, whenever one of us other students presented a case to him during attending rounds, the cardiologist

would berate us, comparing us to Nirenstein, asking why
we couldn't be as smart, as dedicated, as hard-working
as our fellow student.

While Nirenstein sat in his chair smiling smugly, each
of the rest of us, independently, increased the resolve to
kill the guy.

Things changed, however, when the second month of
the rotation began. Having finished his month of service,
the cardiologist was replaced on New Year's Day by Dr.
Dennis Miller, a specialist in gastroenterology. A graduate of Schweitzer and of the residency program at
Jonas Bronck Hospital, Dr. Miller was smart and down-
to-earth, with a cynical sense of humor. He also had a
pretty good understanding of what made people like Phil
Nirenstein tick.

During his first night on call at the beginning of January, Nirenstein and the intern with whom he worked
admitted a thirty-four-year-old man who'd been in excellent health until six days before, when he developed a
case of severe, intractable diarrhea. Although the diarrhea had been accompanied by a low-grade fever, this
Mr. Stevenson had no other symptoms. When he first
developed the diarrhea, Mr. Stevenson hadn't much been
bothered by it. On the afternoon of his admission, after
nearly a week of constant abdominal pain without any
letup, he presented himself to the Jonas Bronck emergency room, where, after a complete evaluation, he was
judged to be more than 7 percent dehydrated. An intravenous line was placed in the patient's arm, through
which a liter of normal saline solution was run, and the
man was admitted to 4 South for further rehydration and
monitoring of his condition.

On hearing of Mr. Stevenson's presence in the emergency room and of his impending admission to the fourth
floor, Nirenstein came very close to having an orgasm.
He understood how critically important this patient could
be to him, how far an outstanding presentation and discussion of the man's disease process would go in im-

pressing Dr. Miller and ensuring himself an honors grade for the month. What better way to get on the good side of a gastroenterologist, Nirenstein reasoned, than to present an old-fashioned case of diarrhea? So, aware of the treasure that lay buried at his feet, Nirenstein plunged into his work.

He ran to the medical library on the third floor of the hospital and quickly read the chapter on diarrheal disease in the most recent edition of Harrison's textbook *Principles of Internal Medicine*. After making a list of all the causes of diarrhea, Nirenstein then checked on as many of the etiologic agents as he could. With this information in hand, feeling as prepared as a heavyweight boxer who has trained for months to fight the champion, Phil Nirenstein went off in search of the new patient.

By the time Nirenstein got to him, Mr. Stevenson must have been feeling much better than he had when he'd first entered the emergency room. Had he still been feeling sick or weak he couldn't possibly have survived the medical student's intensive history-taking session. Nirenstein apparently showed no mercy.

Mr. Stevenson told me later that Nirenstein had pestered him about almost everything. "He was like a defense attorney cross-examining me," the patient said. I imagine their conversation must have gone something like this:

"Have you recently traveled outside the United States?" the medical student asked first.

"Not that I'm aware of," Mr. Stevenson responded.

"You're sure? No trips to Africa or South America, or other places where conditions are primitive?"

"Not that I recall," Mr. Stevenson said. "In fact, I haven't been anywhere outside the United States in years."

"Well, how about travel within the United States? Any trips to rural areas where there are unsanitary conditions?"

"I haven't even left the Bronx in two months," the patient replied. "Not that the Bronx is all that sanitary."

"Well, how about your diet? What did you eat for breakfast three days before you started having the diarrhea?"

"Three days before I started having the diarrhea?" Mr. Stevenson asked, surprised. "You realize that was a week and a half ago, don't you? Do you really expect me to remember what I had for breakfast a week and a half ago?"

"Mr. Stevenson, you have to understand, these questions are very important," the student responded. "You can't expect us to diagnose the cause of your condition unless we have every bit of information possible. Now, please try to remember."

Nirenstein continued. Though he had drawn a blank about that particular breakfast, he relentlessly asked about every other meal Mr. Stevenson had eaten prior to the onset of his symptoms: he wanted to know exactly what the man had eaten, precisely with whom he'd eaten it, and whether anyone else had come down with this or any other type of illness. "In the days before you became sick," Nirenstein urged, "did you eat any raw or poorly cooked shellfish?"

"No." Mr. Stevenson was beginning to lose his patience.

"Are you sure?" Nirenstein said. "No lobster or clams? You're positive about that?"

"I never eat shellfish," the man answered. "I'm allergic."

"Still, no one might have slipped you some? Accidentally, I mean. None of your friends or relatives could possibly have done that?"

"Look, I didn't eat any shellfish, okay?" the man said testily. By now he was getting angry at the badgering. "It would have given me a bad allergy attack and I didn't have any allergy attacks last week."

Giving up on shellfish, Nirenstein pressed on. "How about pork? Any raw or poorly cooked pork?" Mr. Stevenson had not eaten any pork whatsoever.

In the same manner, Nirenstein asked that poor man

about whether he drank unpasteurized cow or goat milk. Going down his list of causes of diarrhea, he quizzed the patient about his work habits, and whether he had recently changed jobs. He inquired about his pets: "Do you keep any pigeons, or chickens, or waterfowl?"

"Right, chickens and waterfowl!" Mr. Stevenson replied, now visibly annoyed. "I have forty chickens and three dozen ducks living in my apartment. This is ridiculous!"

"Look, it may seem ridiculous to you, but it's dead serious," Nirenstein responded, himself becoming annoyed at the patient's attitude. "I'm just trying to do my job. I'm asking these questions to try to help you. I'd appreciate it if you would cooperate. Now, do you keep any pigeons, chickens, or waterfowl?"

"No," Mr. Stevenson tersely replied.

"Any turtles?" the medical student asked. A quizzical look flashed across Mr. Stevenson's face, then he shook his head.

"Any recent visits to pet shops?"

"No," the patient responded again.

On and on it went, Nirenstein continuing to come up with a seemingly unending array of ridiculous questions and Mr. Stevenson, growing angrier and angrier with the medical student's pestering and his disrespectful manner, continuing to answer in short, sharp responses. Eventually, a good hour and a half into the session—around the time Nirenstein got down to a detailed inquisition into the man's sexual habits—the patient called a halt to the questioning. He permitted Nirenstein to perform the briefest of physical examinations, but only after threatening that if the student opened his mouth one more time, Mr. Stevenson was going to call the head nurse and have him thrown out of the hospital.

Nirenstein didn't find anything significant in the physical exam. Since his history, which up to the point when Mr. Stevenson called an abrupt but completely appropriate halt, was completely negative, the student didn't have much to work with. After talking the case over with his intern, the two decided on a plan of action: they'd send off some routine blood work to look for signs of widespread infection, obtain fresh specimens of Mr. Stevenson's stool to examine for the presence of bacteria and parasites, then they'd simply observe the patient while giving him nothing to eat by mouth and keeping him well hydrated with liters of intravenous fluid.

At about three o'clock the next morning, while his intern, who had somehow finished all his work, was off getting a few hours' sleep in the on-call room, Nirenstein slunk back into the library; instead of sleeping, he spent the remaining hours before dawn reading everything he could get his hands on concerning diarrheal disease. By the time the sun rose at a little after six, Nirenstein had stretched his list of causes of acute diarrhea to nearly a hundred separate entities. Satisfied that he had included virtually every possible cause, he then divided his list into three separate categories: those entities that were most likely to have caused Mr. Stevenson's illness, those that were least likely, and those that fell somewhere in between.

Attending rounds began at a little after ten o'clock in the morning. After we'd all taken seats in the staff lounge just off the nurses' station on 4 South, Dr. Miller asked the senior resident if there were any new cases that needed to be discussed. When the resident reported that a Mr. Stevenson had been admitted to the ward after having had diarrhea of unknown etiology for a week, the attending's eyes opened wide. "A GI case," he said in that sardonic tone of his. "How wonderful! Who's the lucky guy who's going to present it?"

Without waiting for an introduction, Nirenstein launched into his presentation. Although he hadn't gotten a wink of sleep the night before, he looked fresh, awake and oriented. Nirenstein had an amazing resiliency: he always managed to look his best, no matter how bad things had been the night before.

Dennis Miller didn't seem overly impressed with Nirenstein's presentation. He interrupted the student more than once, requesting each time that he speed things up. "So what do you think the patient's got?" the attending finally asked, to the delight of the rest of us medical students on the team, well before Nirenstein had even had a chance to get through presenting the findings from his physical examination.

"The most likely cause is infectious," Nirenstein responded, a little disturbed that Dennis Miller didn't seem to be falling for his game plan. Looking down at the list he'd drawn up in the library a few hours before, Nirenstein began to recite a litany of infectious agents that had, at one time or another, been reported to cause diarrhea. He got out at least twenty Latinate names before Dr. Miller interrupted again. "Yeah, yeah, we know all that, but what do you think the guy's got?"

"Well, in light of the high white blood cell count," Nirenstein answered, "and the fact that there's a preponderance of lymphocytes in the differential count, I'd have to put salmonella at the top of the list."

"Salmonella, huh?" the attending replied. "Okay, I'll buy that. I think salmonella's a very good bet. Okay, so let's say this guy does have salmonella. How'd he get it? Has he had any exposure to anything that might carry it?"

"No," Nirenstein said, somewhat defeated. "That's the only trouble. I asked the patient about everything. He hasn't been around anyone who's had diarrhea. He hasn't eaten any raw fish or chicken or meat. He hasn't been on a farm, and he doesn't have any pet turtles."

"Well, there's got to be something," the attending said. "Maybe you missed it."

"No, I don't think I missed anything," Nirenstein asserted, drawing a shake of the head and a cynical leer from the attending. "I asked about all the possible risk factors."

"Well, we'll see," Dennis Miller responded. "Let's go over and talk to the guy."

Together we walked down the hall toward Mr. Stevenson's bed. When we arrived the patient shook hands with Dr. Miller, nodded toward the intern who had admitted him, and sneered toward Nirenstein, who, having shoved his way to the front of the group, was standing directly beside the attending physician. After introducing himself, Dr. Miller asked Mr. Stevenson how he was feeling. "Much better," the patient said.

"I'm glad to hear it," said Dr. Miller. "Listen, this doctor here has been telling me a little about what's been going on with you over the past few days." Mr. Stevenson rolled his eyes when Dr. Miller pointed toward Nirenstein. "He told me you haven't eaten anything new or unusual within the past week or so, is that right?"

"That's absolutely true," Mr. Stevenson replied. "All I've eaten is the same old stuff I've always eaten."

"He said you haven't been around anyone who's been sick?"

"No," the patient said. "Everyone I know has been just fine."

"You haven't taken any trips recently?"

The patient shook his head.

"And nobody in your family has any pets?" Dr. Miller asked.

Mr. Stevenson gazed at the attending with a kind of smile on his face. "I never said that," Mr. Stevenson answered, shaking his head slightly.

"Oh, so you do have pets?" Dr. Miller asked, apparently not very surprised by this disclosure. "What kind?"

"My son's got three tortoises," the man said.

Nirenstein's eyes opened wide and his face turned bright red. "But you told me you didn't have any turtles!" the student said, bewildered.

"We don't have turtles," Mr. Stevenson replied angrily. "We have tortoises. Everybody knows that tortoises are very different from turtles. You don't have to be a genius to know that."

"Have your son's tortoises been in good health recently, Mr. Stevenson?'' the attending asked, trying hard to suppress a laugh.

"Well, no, not really. In fact, until last week we actually had four of them. One day last week, one of them just rolled over and died."

By now all of us were trying to hold ourselves together. All, that is, except Nirenstein, who was glaring hard at the patient. "Why didn't you tell me that?" he shouted at the man. "Why didn't you tell me when I asked you about pets last night? You knew why I was asking those questions!"

"I didn't tell you because you were so damned nasty about the whole thing," the man shouted back. "If you'd have been a nice guy and had asked nicely, like this doctor just did, I would've been glad to tell you about our tortoises. Maybe this'll teach you to be nice to people when they're sick."

After apologizing to the patient for Nirenstein's behavior the night before (while the medical student stood in silence, mortified), Dr. Miller explained what had caused his symptoms. He told Mr. Stevenson that he was most probably suffering from an infection with the bacterium *Salmonella typhi*, that he had probably contracted the infection from his son's dead tortoise, and that he'd probably soon feel well enough to return home. After bidding farewell to the patient, Dr. Miller led us out of the room and back to the lounge.

"So what have we learned from this experience?" the attending asked when we had reclaimed our seats. "As I see it, there are three lessons here. First, we've learned that patients don't like it very much when their doctors act like schmucks and treat them like dirt. Second, we've learned that you can usually get all the information you need by acting like a mensch and being friendly and courteous to the patient. And probably most important, we've learned that turtles are definitely not the same as tortoises."

As expected, the culture taken of Mr. Stevenson's stool specimen grew out a pure colony of *Salmonella typhi*.

The man recovered without incident and was discharged from the hospital three days after he'd first been admitted. Although Phil Nirenstein's behavior became a little less flamboyant over the next few weeks, he never quite recovered from his screw-up on Mr. Stevenson. Having failed to impress Dennis Miller the way he had the cardiologist, Nirenstein had had to settle for a grade of high pass in internal medicine. Phil might have blown his chance of getting a prestigious internship at Mass. General, but he did learn an important lesson in zoology.

As I took a detailed history from Mrs. Iqbal that morning in November 1977, my words may have sounded similar to the ones uttered by Nirenstein in cross-examining Mr. Stevenson the year before, but my patient responded very differently from the way Mr. Stevenson had reacted to my classmate. Throughout, Mrs. Iqbal seemed happy to answer my questions, even the ones that must have seemed irrelevant and silly to her.

"Have you noticed any problems with your eyesight?" I asked at the start of the portion of the history known as the review of systems.

"No, it's about the same as it's always been," she answered.

"Any blurriness of vision?" I went on.

"No."

"Any double-vision?"

She shook her head.

"Have you had any earaches recently?"

"I've never had an earache in my life."

"Any recent problems with your hearing?"

"No, my hearing has been fine."

"Any discharge from your ears?"

Again she shook her head.

"Any problems with your nose, or with your sense of smell?"

Mrs. Iqbal paused and looked thoughtful. "Now that you mention it, there is something about my nose. I've noticed that it looks . . . different."

I wrote this down. "In what way does it look different?" I asked.

"I'm not really sure," she answered. "It's just that lately it seems to have a different shape."

I wrote this down also. "Do you think it's bigger, or maybe a little smaller?" I pressed, having absolutely no idea what any of this might mean.

She considered these options for a few seconds. "No," she said, "it's about the same size. It's hard to explain: it just has a slightly different shape."

After adding this comment to my notes, we went on. The rest of the review of systems, just as ridiculously detailed, revealed nothing helpful. And the physical exam I performed was also pretty much a waste of time; Mrs. Iqbal, though febrile, otherwise appeared to be as healthy as a horse. When my work was completed I thanked her profusely for her patience, shook her hand, and said that I'd be back later in the day with the rest of the infectious disease team.

As I reviewed my notes, trying to develop a list of possible diagnoses that could explain Mrs. Iqbal's symptoms and signs, my brain became fixated on a single disorder: leprosy. For some reason I remembered from my first-year microbiology course, the one I'd failed, something about leprosy causing damage to the structures of the nose. Not able to get this thought out of my head, I went to the hospital library and looked up leprosy in a textbook of medicine; surprisingly, I found that I was correct: infection with the agent that causes leprosy, *Mycobacterium leprae*, can lead to slow but steady changes in the cooler, exposed tissues of the body, including the skin, nose, and eyes. As I read the brief description of the disease, I became convinced that leprosy was the cause of Mrs. Iqbal's symptoms. Sure, the book mentioned that only very rarely had cases of leprosy ever been reported in the United States outside of the Deep South, and that fever, although occasionally present, was not a common feature of the disease. But after all, I reasoned, what else could be responsible for making a patient's nose suddenly change shape? Mrs. Iqbal had leprosy; there was no question about it.

At precisely one P.M. the infectious disease team reassembled in the bacteriology lab to begin daily attending rounds. After introducing himself to us, Dr. Zimmerman, the heavyset, balding director of the lab who would be our attending physician that month, asked Fred Stein if any new cases needed to be discussed. "There's a patient over on 4 East with fever of unknown origin we were asked to consult on," the resident replied. "The medical student saw her this morning." Turning to me, he asked, "Are you ready to present the case?"

I nodded yes, then launched into the story, relying heavily on my pages of notes. About ten minutes into my presentation, Zimmerman, realizing that if he didn't do something soon I would probably spend most of the rest of the afternoon reporting the history I'd obtained, interrupted. "Would you mind limiting your remarks to just the pertinent facts? Don't get me wrong. I really would love to hear more about this woman's first cousin in New Delhi with multiple sclerosis, but we've only got an hour." So I continued on, a little intimidated, mentioning only the information I thought might be considered important.

Twenty minutes later, at the conclusion of my presentation, Dr. Zimmerman, who I'm pretty sure had nodded off to sleep sometime between his comment to me and my description of Mrs. Iqbal's physical exam, suddenly came back to life. "So what do you think she's got?"

I paused a moment for dramatic effect. And then, proudly, I replied: "Leprosy."

The attending's eyes opened wide, but his stunned silence lasted for only a brief second; then both he and Fred Stein burst into chuckles. Their laughter steadily grew more and more raucous until I became concerned that the attending physician might fall out of his chair. Only as the guffawing began to abate, as Zimmerman was wiping the tears from his eyes, sighing, "Where the hell do they *find* these medical students?'' did I begin to have some serious reservations about the likelihood of my primary diagnosis. ''Leprosy, that's great,'' Zimmerman finally said. ''What makes you think she's got leprosy?''

''Well, she's had this fever,'' I answered tentatively, ''and she says her nose looks different. What else could it be?''

My response caused more howls of laughter to be released from both the resident and the attending. ''What else could it be?'' Zimmerman repeated when he regained control of himself. ''That's terrific.''

''It's like the Tsutsugamushi fever joke,'' Fred said, reciting the name, I was to discover later, of an exceedingly rare form of typhus. ''Patient comes into the emergency room complaining of fever and diarrhea. The medical student examines the guy and makes a tentative diagnosis of Tsutsugamushi fever. The patient gets admitted, and sure enough, the workup shows the guy does have Tsutsugamushi fever. The chief resident comes up to the student, very impressed, and says, 'Gee, that was amazing. What ever tipped you off to the fact that this guy had Tsutsugamushi?' And the student says, 'What else causes fever and diarrhea?' ''

This story produced more peals of laughter from Zimmerman, who was now doubled over and grabbing at his meaty flanks. ''We've got to stop this,'' he choked out, ''or I'm going to wet my pants. We'd better go down to the ward and have a look at your leper.''

By the time we reached 4 East, Dr. Zimmerman had brought himself under control again. He was very polite when he introduced himself to Mrs. Iqbal, asking her to recite again, briefly, her symptoms. After performing a cursory physical examination and then thanking the patient for her cooperation, the attending physician led us out of the isolation room. Once we were out in the hall he began giving his discourse: ''Needless to say, the differential diagnosis of fever of unknown origin is tremendously long.'' He then rambled through a discussion of some of the more common entities which needed to be considered in the patient, both those caused by infectious agents and those completely unrelated to infections. He did mention leprosy, but it was way down at the very bottom of his list. And then, looking directly at me with a gleam in his eye, Zimmerman asked, "Do you have any idea when the last case of leprosy was diagnosed in the Bronx?" When I failed to reply, the attending continued: "It's been years and years. I do have to admit that it is on the differential diagnosis list, but I'm so sure that this woman doesn't have it that I'll make a deal with you: if this patient turns out to have leprosy and you can prove it, I'll give you a grade of honors for the month."

Okay, so maybe it was a ridiculous idea, but now he'd done it. Zimmerman had thrown down the academic gauntlet, and I had no choice but to accept the challenge. Like Phil Nirenstein, most students at Schweitzer would literally kill for a grade of honors in nearly any clinical rotation, and I was certainly no exception. The only thing standing between me and a grade of honors in this elective was proving that Mrs. Iqbal had leprosy. And so I set to work.

Through reading, I found out that the only way to make a positive diagnosis of leprosy was to grow *Mycobacterium leprae* from skin scrapings taken from the patient's most involved area. No one at Jonas Bronck Hospital knew of a facility in the Bronx or anywhere else where cultures of this bacterium could be grown. In desperation, I contacted the New York City Department of Health in Manhattan, and one of the staff members there gave me the telephone number of a laboratory at the Centers for Disease Control in Atlanta. The lab kept armadillos, the only animals other than human beings in which the bacterium will grow. I arranged with one of the hospital administrators to have the samples shipped, collected dozens of skin scrapings from the region around Mrs. Iqbal's nose, boxed the samples myself, and sat back, waiting for the call back from Georgia.

* * *

The month passed fairly rapidly. I learned very little about infectious diseases, but I did figure out the importance of keeping one's mouth shut during attending rounds and not being overly enthusiastic about offering opinions on patients' diagnoses. One afternoon, Mrs. Iqbal's fever vanished just as mysteriously as it had appeared, and it didn't return. The woman was discharged from the hospital on November 13, with an appointment to be seen the following week in one of the outpatient clinics. By the last week of the month I'd nearly forgotten about the whole incident. But then, on the next-to-last day of the rotation, Dr. Zimmerman appeared for attending rounds with a dazed look on his face. "I can't believe it!" he said, staring in my direction. "I just got off the phone with the director of the *Mycobacterium* lab at the CDC. He said the preliminary cultures have confirmed the growth of *Mycobacterium leprae* in the skin scrapings from that Mrs. Iqbal."

A smile cracked across my face. "You mean she actually has leprosy?" Fred Stein asked with amazement. Our attending nodded.

It took a while before I could get the words out. "So that means I get honors, right?"

"I guess so," Zimmerman replied. "I still can't believe it myself. Fever's not even a major symptom of leprosy. Amazing."

It has often been said by critics of medical education that far too much time in medical school is spent on the rarities of medicine rather than the common disorders that afflict patients. These critics contend that when students hear hoofbeats coming down the street outside the buildings of the medical school, it's been hammered into them to think of zebras instead of horses (or, in the case of Phil Nirenstein, to dwell on turtles instead of tortoises). That criticism might often be valid, but in the Bronx, where just about anything can happen, this philosophy of education actually makes a great deal of sense. After all, there aren't many horses around anymore, and what with the Bronx Zoo being so close by, zebras aren't all that rare.

By the time I started that elective rotation in infectious diseases in November 1977, I had made my final decision about specialization: I would spend my career working in pediatrics. During the nearly one and a half years since I'd first set foot on the wards of Jonas Bronck Hospital I had been drawn to pediatrics. First, as opposed to internal medicine, where the majority of patients seemed to suffer from unremitting, incurable, chronic diseases, nearly all the children who came to the hospital for medical care completely recovered from their illnesses and contributing to this recovery was gratifying. Next, watching healthy children grow and develop was actually fun—certainly more enjoyable than witnessing the slow but steady deterioration of patients in most other medical specialties. And finally, the persons with whom I had worked in the pediatric department at Schweitzer, from the lowliest intern to the most senior attending physician, were the friendliest and most humanistic of all the medical personnel I'd interacted with since beginning my rotations on the wards. Pediatricians seemed concerned not just with their patients' medical needs, but with their social and psychological requirements as well. My decision to become a pediatrician wasn't all that difficult to make.

And so, in late September I wrote away to ten pediatric programs in the northeastern United States, requesting applications for an internship position beginning in July 1978. I also petitioned the medical school to allow me to do my two-month subinternship, a rotation during which the senior medical student works as an intern, in pediatrics. My petition was approved, and I spent December of that year working in the neonatal intensive care unit at Jonas Bronck Hospital.

5

My First Night on Call in the Intensive Care Unit from Hell

Subinternship in neonatal ICU, December 1977

In December of my senior year I elected to spend a month working as a subintern in the neonatal intensive care unit at Jonas Bronck Hospital. Looking back on that decision, I realize that I must have been out of my mind. The NICU had always been the most difficult rotation, both technically and emotionally, in the pediatric residency training program at Jonas Bronck Hospital. The unit, home to between twenty and thirty of the sickest, tiniest, most medically demanding premature infants, was a nightmarish place to work, a ward that through the years had come to be known to the interns and residents forced to spend a month or two working there as the Intensive Care Unit from Hell. It took me only one night to understand why.

I started December with three strikes against me. First, I had no idea of what to do, or even how to act, around these minuscule infants; in all the time I'd spent in medical school, not only had I never been permitted to enter the NICU, I hadn't even ever seen a premature infant up close. Second, I had developed none of the technical skills needed for working in the unit. Although I was by then competent in drawing blood from adult veins, I had little chance of being able to start an intravenous line, perform a spinal tap, or get blood from an infant as tiny as the ones who inhabited the NICU. Finally, I had never before been the primary caretaker of any hospitalized patient, young or old. As I passed through the unit's electric doors at seven-thirty on the first Monday morning in December, leaving behind the world of just plain Jonas Bronck Hospital and entering the high-tech wonderland that was the NICU, I was, to say the least, scared shitless.

"There's nothing to worry about," Jonathan Simon, the neonatologist in charge of the unit, told me when I expressed my fears to him in his office during the short orientation session that preceded my first morning of work. "When you see them for the first time, the babies might look a little frightening to you, but you'll get over that pretty quickly. And once you've been working for a day or two, I'm sure you'll get the hang of the place. But even if you don't, and it does happen to take you a little longer than that to adjust, don't worry about a thing: you're never going to find yourself alone in my unit. There'll always be the senior resident or at least one of the interns around to help you out. The house staff will make sure you don't wind up completely screwing things up."

My talk with Dr. Simon reassured me, at least temporarily; but then we started rounds.

We began in the first of five rooms, each about fifteen feet square, that comprised the patient care area of the unit. NICU-Room I, where the sickest infants were housed, was at maximum capacity that morning, its facilities taken up by five objects that Jonathan Simon repeatedly referred to as our patients. The bodies of these patients, who to me looked more like undercooked chicken wings needing at least another hour in the oven before they'd be ready to eat than like human babies, were laid out on separate warming tables, tiny mattresses enclosed in collapsible Plexiglas frames under heat-radiating overhead canopies. Each infant was virtually encased in monitor leads, wires, and tubing attached to what appeared to be dozens of complicated, expensive, and (at least to me) utterly incomprehensible machines. Because of respiratory distress syndrome, a serious lung disease that occurs in premature babies, each of the infants in NICU-Room I that morning required the assistance of a mechanical ventilator in order to get enough oxygen into its lungs. The loud, repetitive siss pump—siss pump—siss pump sounds coming from the five ventilators made it nearly impossible to hear anything else, including normal human conversation, while standing in that room.

Despite the noise, Dr. Simon spent the next hour hanging in turn over each baby's bedside, spouting off details about each patient's condition as loud as he could. I understood not a single sentence he said. At first I thought that because of the din made by the ventilators I was missing a key word or two out of every ten the attending emitted. But then, after I got up close to the doctor and tried my best to concentrate on every word he said, I realized that the problem was more than just the noise of the machines: using abbreviations, mysterious-sounding words, and phrases that didn't make any sense at all, the attending was speaking in what amounted to a foreign language, one I'd never heard before. "Since this baby's pO_2 is only forty-eight, it's pretty clear we're going to have to go up on some setting or other," he said matter-of-factly as we stood over the warming table of the first patient, a child who, having weighed only slightly more than a pound at birth, had been hovering near death during every moment of the two weeks that had thus far composed his life. "Since the FiO_2 is already up to a hundred, we're going to have to crank up either the pressure or the rate. Since the rate's already up to forty and I don't feel comfortable going any higher than that, let's try increasing the PEEP; I'll turn it up to twenty-four, and we'll see what happens."

What happened was simple: I became completely and hopelessly lost, unable to figure out what the hell was going on with any of these tiny, unfortunate babies. It quickly became clear that Dr. Simon's prediction of my being able to get the hang of working in the NICU in a day or two was more than a little optimistic; a more realistic estimate was a year or two. Resigning myself to the fact that understanding any of this neonatology stuff in the time allotted for the subinternship was utterly hopeless, I saw that I would have to alter my objectives radically: rather than attempting to master neonatology, I decided that just getting through the month without killing anyone would be a more appropriate goal. I thus tried to take comfort in the second part of Dr. Simon's pep talk, his guarantee that there would always be someone else around, the resident or one of the three interns, to protect these semihuman creatures who were our patients from any harm I might inadvertently cause them. But then, during that first day, I came to know a little more about the resident and interns.

The house officers who were assigned to work in the NICU that month happened to be the four most incompetent, most hopelessly confused physicians the Jonas Bronck pediatric residency program at that time employed. Throughout the year they had each managed, in ways uniquely their own, to endanger the lives of the patients entrusted to their care and to infuriate the rest of the house staff. By some horrendous quirk of scheduling fate, against odds that must have been astronomical, all four had been brought together that month to work on the single most demanding rotation at Jonas Bronck Hospital. And, lucky me, I'd chosen that same month to do an elective with them.

Clearly the worst of the interns was a man who had applied for his internship position as Jack, a normal, sensitive senior student from a medical school in upstate New York who had apparently truly wanted to be a pediatrician at one time. But sometime between the day he filed his application for the job and the day he showed up for orientation, Jack had been transformed into Yitzhak, a devout Lubavitcher, a member of a Jewish sect so orthodox, so ultra-observant, that his beliefs precluded him from working on Friday nights, Saturdays, and holidays. These restrictions required that Yitzhak make extensive changes in the every-third-night-on-call work schedule. At the beginning of his internship year he had tried to convince the chief residents, who made up the monthly schedules, to work these problems out for him. They gave it their best shot, but after only one month—when they began to realize what a massive headache would result from trying to keep everybody involved happy—they told the born-again Lubavitcher that he'd have to work out the details of such an arrangement on his own. Yitzhak had tried to trade slots in the schedule with his fellow interns in each successive rotation and, as a result, had gotten into argument after argument with nearly every one of them, for they were of course reluctant to sacrifice their free Friday or Saturday nights to cover for him. Yitzhak's persistence, and his anger whenever anyone refused to cooperate with his demands, had caused widespread resentment within the residency program.

Others might have been more sympathetic to his plight if Yitzhak had at least occasionally been willing to pitch in and fulfill his responsibilities. But unlike his earlier incarnation as Jack, he no longer seemed to want to be a doctor at all; he now wanted to be a Talmudic scholar. During the time he spent in the hospital, Yitzhak performed almost no patient care. When he should have been working either he could be found sitting in the nurses' station, pulling at his scraggly, unkempt red beard and mustache while he read from the holy books he kept in his locker in the residents' room, or he wasn't to be found at all. Before his frequent periods of absence, Yitzhak would tell the nurses that he was going off to pray; sometimes these private prayer sessions would last for hours.

The second intern on our team that month was Sharon, a well-meaning but completely overwhelmed woman whose problems transcended the typical hardships inherent in internship, penetrating deep into her personal life. Already on a shaky foundation at the start of her internship year, Sharon's fragile marriage had been unable to withstand the rigors of the on-call schedule and the chronic exhaustion that it produced. And so, one day after an especially difficult night on call in September, Sharon returned home from work to find that her husband, without a word or even a note, had packed up and left their apartment. Then, in the middle of November, just when she'd begun to recover a little from the breakup of her marriage, her mother, after a battle with breast cancer that had gone on for more than five years, took a turn for the worse and died. Sharon was trying to work through these tragedies, but by December she was finding it more and more difficult to carry on.

Near the end of rounds on that first morning, more than two hours after I had tuned out the proceedings and begun to calculate the number of days I would be on duty until the month came to an end, Dr. Simon reprimanded Sharon for forgetting to order an X ray he had requested the day before on one of her healthier patients. The neonatologist was gentle in his criticism, but Sharon was nearly in tears. After rounds ended I walked into the nurses' station and found Sharon sitting on the floor, performing some sort of operation on the wheels of the transport incubator, the device used to carry sick newborns from the delivery room to the NICU. Figuring that this was one of the routine tasks I too would be expected to perform, I asked her what she was doing.

"I'm pulling lint out of the wheels," she replied seriously without looking up, concentrating all her attention on the pair of tweezers in her right hand as they grabbed between the wheels for another payload. "You know, hair and stuff gets caught down there, and sometimes it's hard to get the wheels to turn right."

I looked on, amazed, watching her silently attack each of the four wheels until Mary, the head nurse of the unit during the day shift, tapped me on the shoulder and gestured for me to join her out in the hall. When we were far enough away so that Sharon couldn't overhear, the nurse told me what was really going on: "Don't worry, you're not going to have to do that," she told me, apparently reading my mind. "That's just something Sharon does whenever someone yells at her. Anytime something goes wrong or one of her patients gets sick or something like that she takes out those tweezers, sits right down on the floor, and starts working on the transporter."

"It sounds pretty weird," I replied. "Is it, like, some form of therapy?"

"I guess," Mary said. "We're all really worried about her. That's not a normal way to act."

The final intern on our team was Jennifer, an intelligent, competent woman who, during the course of the half year since she'd entered the residency program had simply burned out. During rounds on that first day she stood silently, away from our little group, volunteering no information about her patients unless directly asked by Dr. Simon. I tried to make small talk with her during that morning, but she completely ignored me. Clearly Jennifer didn't want to have anything to do with me, with the other interns, residents, and attendings, or, most disturbing, with her patients.

What these three interns needed was a strong, dominating senior resident who could take charge and put them all on the proper course. What they got, unfortunately for all of us, was Manny Vasquez.

Even as a third-year medical student, a position well out of the mainstream of hospital life, I had heard rumors about Manny. The stories were repeated so many times that they had almost become part of the hospital's folklore. They revolved around allegations that, in addition to being a pediatric resident nearing the end of his three years of training, Manny was also a major Bronx drug dealer. Various accounts had him either directly selling drugs that had been stolen from the hospital pharmacy or simply selling prescriptions, signed and completed with his official Drug Enforcement Agency authorization number, to the janitors, food service workers, and other hospital employees from a rarely used storage closet in the subbasement of Jonas Bronck Hospital. Supposedly the hospital administrators knew all about Manny's sideline business but were keeping the details quiet so as to circumvent the community outrage that might erupt if Manny were disciplined: born in Puerto Rico and raised in the south Bronx, Manny was a genuine success story in our area, a ghetto kid who had overcome tremendous adversity and finally made it. He was a role model for many of the children, mostly from Hispanic backgrounds, who came to our hospital's pediatric clinics and emergency room. News that Manny was involved in criminal activities, especially drug-related criminal activities, could have had a devastating effect on community relations. Manny had therefore been quietly talked to and the whole thing was forgotten, but the activities, it was said, continued.

On beginning my rotation in the NICU I didn't know for sure whether these stories about Manny were true or not, but I did find out soon enough that the senior resident spent a lot of time away from the unit, which meant that his interns had to rely on their own resources. This was the resident who, according to Jonathan Simon, was going to make sure I didn't make a complete fool of myself.

I found myself on call the very first night of my rotation in the neonatal intensive care unit. The evening started off relatively quietly; the first part of it I spent sitting in the interns' on-call room, located just down the hall from the NICU. I told the nurses I'd be reading, but what I was really doing was trying my best to hide. Things had been going smoothly and I hadn't been disturbed even once until, at about eleven-thirty, a newborn was transferred to the unit from Jefferson Hospital, a small hospital in the west Bronx which had no neonatal intensive care unit. According to the history given by the physician who had accompanied the baby in the ambulance, the infant had been born without complications but, about two hours after birth, had had what appeared to be a prolonged convulsion. The doctors at Jefferson, uncomfortable to have responsibility for a child with so potentially serious a problem, had called for an ambulance and shipped the baby to Jonas Bronck for evaluation and treatment.

I came out of the on-call room to meet the ambulance team when the baby arrived in the NICU. After helping some of the night shift nurses transfer the child to one of the warming tables in NICU–Room 2, I watched as they went through the ritual of admitting a newborn to the unit: the nurses weighed the infant and measured his length, judging him to be appropriately grown for a full-term infant. They measured his head circumference, which was found to be pretty normal as well. Then they covered him with the network of monitor leads, wires, and tubing I had earlier noted surrounding the other babies in the unit. When the nurses were done with him, Annette, the head nurse on the night shift, turned to me and said, "Well, Doc, what do you want to do?"

At first I was confused by this question, but then, when I realized she was talking to me, I carefully explained that I was no doctor, that I was only a fourth-year medical student doing an elective rotation, and that I didn't know anything about what needed to be done for this, or for that matter, for any of the other critically ill babies in the unit. "Maybe you'd better call for some help," Annette suggested.

That seemed like a good idea. I went out to the nurses' station and called the page operator, asking her to page Manny Vasquez, who was on call with me that night. I then sat back and waited for the phone to ring. Fifteen minutes had passed by the time Annette, who'd been busy with the new arrival, came and asked, "Well, what should we do? Do you want to start an IV?"

"I don't know," I replied. "Manny hasn't called back yet."

"When did you page him?"

"About fifteen minutes ago."

"Well, he's not going to call back," she said. "When was the last time you saw him?"

"Around seven o'clock. He said he had some stuff to take care of, but if I needed him he'd be—"

" 'Right at the end of my beeper, babe' ? "

"Yeah. How did you know?"

"That's what he tells everybody right before he disappears," Annette said. "That means he's gone. We might not see him again for the rest of the night. Who's the intern on with you tonight?"

"Yitzhak," I answered. "He said he'd be off—"

"Praying?" she interrupted again.

"Yeah." I suddenly felt very uneasy.

"Well, that means he's gone too. It looks like you're in charge, Doc." And then she asked that question again: "What do you want to do?"

What I wanted to do, understanding that I might well be the closest thing resembling a doctor working in the NICU that night, was run back to my apartment, crawl under the bed, and hide until the next morning. But instead, I decided to ask for any help I could get. "What should I do?" I asked the nurse.

"Maybe first you should examine the baby," she replied, "and see if you can find anything obvious wrong. Then I guess you're going to have to decide whether you want to treat the kid with seizure medication or not."

It sounded like a logical plan, so I followed as Annette led me back into NICU–Room 2. "I can't do any harm examining him," I thought, and I prayed that by the time I had finished the exam either Manny or Yitzhak would have shown up. So I slowly began to look the infant over.

I had spent most of my first afternoon in the NICU hanging out with Jennifer, who, although obviously very depressed, was the only one of the three interns who still seemed to have any sense about her; I figured that if I watched her closely I could at least fake my way through some of the things that were expected of me. Although Jennifer was not exactly ecstatic about having me shadow her every move, she had allowed me to tag along as long as I promised not to ask any questions—or for that matter, carry on any conversation with her at all. During the afternoon I'd watched her perform physical exams on normal newborns in the well-baby nursery, and now, faced with the baby from Jefferson Hospital, I did everything I had seen her do earlier in the day: I measured the baby's length and his head circumference; I checked his eyes with a bright light; I noted that he had two each of eyes, ears, arms, and legs; I counted a total of twenty fingers and toes; using my stethoscope, I listened to his heart and lungs; I squeezed his belly and tried to percuss his liver. I had no idea of the significance of my findings; Jennifer hadn't discussed any of that part of the examination with me. Still, I did what I thought was a thorough job, the whole exam taking a little over half an hour. But when I was finished I found that I was still on my own.

Annette came looking for me again at about one o'clock. I was sitting in the nurses' station, working on a very detailed admission note for the chart on the baby from Jefferson Hospital. Annette sat down next to me and said, "Look, I understand the situation you're in, but somebody's got to take charge here. A doctor's got to make a decision about this baby. We can't just let him lie out there, waiting for something to happen. Do you want us to give him some medication or not?"

I said I'd get back to her in a few minutes. I picked up the phone, called the operator again, and asked her to page both Manny and Yitzhak, stat. That was the entire repertoire of what I knew how to do; I didn't even have the sense or smarts to try to phone the neonatal fellow, or the neurologist on call, or Jonathan Simon at home; I didn't even know that I could try to get help from the senior resident on call on the general pediatric ward, who at that moment, I later learned, was sitting in the residents' room, a little more than a hundred yards away from the NICU. I didn't know, and I didn't think, and I shouldn't have been there by myself, alone with all those sick babies. But I was.

When fifteen more minutes had passed and neither

Manny nor Yitzhak had responded to the stat pages, when I could feel Annette starting to inch her way back toward the nurses' station, I bolted. I ran down the hall and into the interns' on-call room, turning off the lights, getting into bed, and pretending to go to sleep. But I could have no sooner slept than I could have made an intelligent decision about whether or not to give that baby seizure medication.

It was about two o'clock in the morning when the alarm in the on-call room went off. I didn't know exactly what the loud, harsh, ringing noise meant, but I knew it had to be trouble, so I got up and quickly made my way back down the hall. Annette and the other night nurses were standing around the baby from Jefferson. When I entered the room the head nurse said, "He just had another seizure. It looks like it stopped on its own, but we can't wait around any longer. This baby's got to get some medicine to stop his seizures or he might die."

I nodded. Annette was right; there was no other possible answer. I had to figure out what kind of anticonvulsant to use on the baby and what dose to give. Without anyone around to help me through, I realized I was going to have to teach myself something about neonatalogy, and that I was going to have to do it in a hurry. Running again into the nurses' station, I looked up the dose of phenobarbital, the only anticonvulsant I knew anything about, in one of the textbooks of neonatology. Reading the whole section on use of the drug, I soon realized that I was in deep trouble: the book said that, in order to prevent seizures in a newborn, phenobarbital had to be given intravenously. "Can you start an IV on this kid?" I asked Annette. When the nurse shook her head I said, "Well, then, we're back to square one." And I went to stat page the intern and resident again.

While I was talking to the page operator, Annette came running in. "He's seizing again," she shouted. I slammed down the phone and ran after her into the baby's room. He was in the midst of a generalized tonic-clonic seizure; his arms and legs were shaking and his eyes had rolled back in their sockets. The convulsion continued on and on. The nurses and I stood by, helplessly, watching the baby convulse and listening as the *beep beep beep* sounds coming from his cardiac monitor gradually slowed from 140 beeps a minute to less than 100 to less than 50. As we stood there, the baby from Jefferson Hospital died before our eyes.

We tried to resuscitate him, but it was hopeless. With no IV in place, we couldn't give him any medications to make his heart beat any better or for any longer. I pounded on his chest awhile to try to get the heart pumping again once it had stopped, but it didn't do any good. That poor baby never had a chance.

I declared him dead at about two-thirty in the morning; declaring him dead didn't require any special skill or expertise. I was frightened and disgusted, but mostly I was shocked; I knew that because of my incompetence, my ignorance, and my lack of resourcefulness, I had been responsible for the baby's death. Afterward I slunk back to the bed in the on-call room. Although I didn't sleep a wink, the nurses, mercifully, didn't disturb me for the rest of the night.

The next morning, when Jonathan Simon heard from the nurses the story of the death of the baby from Jefferson Hospital, the attending physician went absolutely nuts. Manny Vasquez, who, as Annette had predicted, had been absent from the unit the entire night, appeared in the morning, acting as if nothing had happened, just in time to start work rounds. Confronting him right in the middle of the NICU–Room I, in front of the whole staff of nurses and doctors, the neonatal attending laid the blame for the baby's death squarely on the shoulders of the senior resident, accusing him of malpractice and telling him that he'd do everything in his power to have the resident's medical license revoked. "You are not fit to practice medicine," the attending shouted at the resident near the end of his tirade, before he threw Manny out of the NICU, warning him never to pass through its doors again.

Dr. Simon tried to make good on his threat to have Manny's medical license revoked, but he came up against resistance from the administration, which wanted to prevent bad blood between the hospital and the community at all costs. The directors of the pediatric department, however, who had been covering up for Manny for two and a half years, had finally had enough, and they took steps to ensure that nothing like the incident that had occurred during that night in December would ever happen again. First, they barred the senior resident from all inpatient responsibilities for the remainder of his training; next, because enough evidence had been accumulated that not only was Manny selling drugs but that he'd also developed a pretty serious addiction to cocaine, the program directors forced the resident into a drug treatment program; and finally, following his seemingly successful completion of the treatment program, Manny was reluctantly permitted to finish his senior residency year in the well-child clinics, where the patients weren't critically ill and his responsibility could not cause significant damage.

After he had completed the year, Manny disappeared. Since then rumors about him have continued to swirl around Jonas Bronck Hospital. One account had him dying of a knife wound suffered during a fight in a bar in Texas, a confrontation that was apparently drug-related. According to another he was rehabilitated, drug-free, and practicing general pediatrics somewhere in the Los Angeles area. Whether either of these stories is true has never been verified; what is clear, however, is that Manuel Vasquez never again set foot within the confines of Jonas Bronck Hospital.

Yitzhak, absent, like Manny, during that entire on-call night, also miraculously reappeared the next morning, just in time for work rounds to begin. But during the confrontation at the beginning of rounds, Dr. Simon did not direct his anger at the intern. Such action would have been pointless: since the start of his internship, Yitzhak's mind had been on subjects far less mundane than the life and death of a newborn infant.

Yitzhak was allowed to continue his rotation in the neonatal intensive care unit, but after that night he was never given any real responsibility. The work he should have been assigned was performed instead by a pediatric nurse practitioner who had been specially hired on very short notice to pick up the slack that had developed in the NICU that month. Less than five weeks after our rotation in the NICU ended, Yitzhak, not unexpectedly, quit medicine altogether. He emigrated to Israel, where he immersed himself full-time in the study of Talmud. Since his departure no news or rumors concerning Yitzhak's postinternship life, unlike Manny's, have filtered back to Jonas Bronck Hospital. I sometimes wonder if, during the long periods of time Yitzhak must spend buried in deep philosophical thought, his mind ever wanders back to that infant from Jefferson Hospital who died one night when he should have been working in the neonatal intensive care unit.

I myself certainly think about that baby a lot, thoughts that even today cause beads of sweat to appear on my forehead. It doesn't help to know that an autopsy revealed that the infant had hydrancephaly, a rare congenital malformation of the brain in which the cerebral hemispheres completely fail to develop. In the intervening years I've tried again and again to convince myself that my complete lack of competence that night made no appreciable difference—that in fact I did the child and his family a favor since even if he had survived, a hydrancephalic baby would have had virtually no chance of leading anything like a normal life. But these silent arguments with myself have been useless; I know that that child died because of me, because I was the only one there, a fourth-year medical student with very little practical experience, very little common sense, and almost no knowledge about the way hospitals operate.

After rounds that morning Dr. Simon took me aside

and calmly, without any hint of reproach in his voice, explained that, if I were ever again to find myself alone in the NICU with no backup from the medical staff, I should call him at home immediately. Sadly, I listened to his speech, not saying a word. I didn't have to say anything; he and I had both learned a tough lesson during my first night on call in the Intensive Care Unit from Hell.

PART II

Internship

candidate makes a positive impression and has good enough credentials the job is offered, and the applicant can then either accept or reject the offer. But this simple system, which has been good enough for American business for centuries, is apparently much too straightforward to use in employing interns. Another, more complicated and tortuous technique had to be developed for medical school graduates; and thus, sometime during the late twentieth century, the system of the Internship Match was created.

The way the Match works is simple in outline. In January of senior year, after interviewing at all the programs to which they have applied, medical students each submit a list of those programs, ranked from first to last choice, to the National Internship and Residency Matching Program (NIRMP). Simultaneously, every hospital in the United States which has a residency program submits a list of all senior medical school students who have applied for positions, similarly ranking the applicants from most to least desirable. Once these lists are received, the information is fed into NIRMP's mainframe computer and the machine couples applicants and programs.

One might think that the matching procedure would end with a friendly letter being mailed from NIRMP Central and received privately by the senior medical student a few days later. But no, a system so benign could not possibly be used for future interns. Instead, the results of the computer's match are printed and stored in vaults at NIRMP Central, then released simultaneously to medical schools and residency programs on the third Wednesday in March. On the afternoon of that day, all across the country, senior medical students are assembled in large lecture halls and the envelopes bearing their hospital assignments for the next year are distributed agonizingly slowly, one by one. At more than a hundred American medical schools, the process is exactly the same: a name is called; the student rises and tentatively approaches the front of the room; the envelope is handed over by the person, usually a dean, who has been entrusted with maintaining the rituals of the Match; the envelope is cautiously opened, and the student either breathes a great sigh of relief because he's matched to his top choice and his dreams have been fulfilled, or he lapses into a terrifying anxiety attack because he's gotten into his third, or fourth, or, God forbid, fifth or sixth choice and the student promptly concludes that his life is ruined.

Such attacks are fueled by students' appreciation of the most nefarious feature of the Match: unlike normal job offers, Match assignments are unconditionally and irrevocably binding. Unless there are extraordinary extenuating circumstances, a student has absolutely no chance of transferring to another program once an assignment to a hospital has been made. So as the dean of academic affairs entered the hall, took his place at the podium, and without any introductory remarks began calling off, in random order, the names of my classmates, I prayed that my dreams would be realized—that, when I tore open the flap of my envelope, the name printed on the sheet inside would be one of the two pediatric programs in Boston to which I had applied.

Despite my experiences in Jonas Bronck Hospital's Intensive Care Unit from Hell, I moved ahead with my plans to become a pediatrician. After returning my applications, I was offered interviews at hospitals in Boston, New York, Philadelphia, and Washington, D.C. And after interviewing at all those places, I chose the programs located in America's medical training Mecca, Boston, Massachusetts, as my first and second choices.

My decision to try for Boston was based largely on advice given to me by my faculty adviser at Schweitzer, a pediatrician named William Kelly. "It probably doesn't really matter where you do your training," Dr. Kelly told me during the meeting we'd had in early September. "The education you'll get will be pretty much the same wherever you go. But to me, it's not a great idea to do your internship and residency at the same place where you went to medical school. If you decide to stay at Schweitzer, you'll wind up learning only the Schweitzer way of thinking about pediatrics. If you go elsewhere, you'll learn a second approach to patient care. That way you can decide which works best and make an intelligent choice about how you want to practice pediatrics. Does that make sense?"

It did make sense. Dr. Kelly also told me first to decide in which city I'd like to live, then to apply to the best programs available in that city.

Dr. Kelly's advice about leaving New York for my internship and residency sounded reasonable. In fact, I had only one problem with it, but that problem was logistically immense: my wife, Beth, still a graduate student in molecular biology at Columbia, wasn't anywhere near the completion of her lab work at the time I was applying for internships. Beth estimated that, after my graduation from medical school, she'd have at least another full year of bench research before she could even think about starting to write her dissertation. And since she couldn't transfer to another school smack in the middle of her research project, my leaving New York to do my internship would mean yet another year of separation for us.

So before I sent out my first application, Beth and I had had some long and serious discussions. After we'd argued the issue back and forth, each of us coming up with pros and cons, we ultimately made the decision that living in different cities was something we could handle. Beth would stay in New York, working to complete her lab project as quickly as possible, while, if I got in, I'd go up to Boston. "What's the big deal?" Beth asked late one night in October. "Two nights out of every three you'll either be in the hospital working your ass off or asleep at home, so tired and grumpy that nobody in their right mind would want to have anything to do with you. And anyway, we'll see each other every weekend: either I'll come up to see you, or you'll come down to see me. I don't see what the big problem is."

I couldn't argue with her. During the early fall of 1977

I therefore interviewed at Boston's two best pediatric internship programs. Without much difficulty I ranked them first and second and in January submitted my final list to NIRMP. The time since then I had spent nervously waiting to see what would happen.

My tense wait did not come to an end until the names of nearly three quarters of my classmates had been called. I watched the little dramas play themselves out at the front of the lecture hall, my anxiousness increasing with each passing minute. Finally my name was called. I rose from my seat, walked carefully to the front of the auditorium, was handed the envelope with my name typed across the front, and then, cautiously, tore its flap open. My spirits rose when I saw the words BOSTON MEDICAL CENTER–PEDIATRICS on the paper inside the envelope. I had gotten my wish; although the program at the Boston Medical Center had been my second choice, I would still be spending the next year in Boston.

7

In the Car at the Airport

**First month of internship,
July 1978**

By concentrating all my efforts, I managed to finish the morning scut work by eight o'clock. While going about my chores, my exhausted mind continued to focus on one single fact: I needed to get out of there. I needed to get out of that neonatal intensive care unit or I would die. I had already begun to develop troubling symptoms: my breathing had become labored; I was inhaling and exhaling at least twice as rapidly as normal; my head was spinning and my belly aching. And these symptoms were growing worse with each passing moment. To save my life I had to get onto the street and breathe fresh nonhospital air as quickly as possible. So as soon as Terry Costa, the intern assigned to the next twenty-four-hour shift appeared at the front door of the NICU at a little after eight o'clock that morning, I approached her with an enormous sense of relief.

''Congratulations,'' Terry said, smiling slightly as she walked briskly into the nurses' station. ''You survived. You officially made it to your first weekend.''

''Oh, yeah, it's Saturday,'' I answered with all the strength I could muster. ''Terrific.'' And with that, I burst into tears.

* * *

I had just finished the first night on call of my internship. During the month of July 1978 I had been farmed out, sent to do my required one-month rotation in the neonatal intensive care unit at St. Anne's Medical Center, a women's hospital in South Boston which was affiliated with the Boston Medical Center. So far the experience had been utterly horrible. Although my subinternship in the NICU at Jonas Bronck Hospital during my senior year of medical school had familiarized me with the language of neonatology and with the sight of the frightening-looking, minuscule preemies who inhabited such places, the St. Anne's NICU made the Jonas Bronck Intensive Care Unit from Hell seem like a friendly neighborhood day-care center.

This NICU was a nightmare. A tertiary-care referral center, it was a place to which sick and dying premature infants were transferred from all over New England, where children born months too soon would either be saved and ultimately, after weeks and weeks of expensive, intensive treatment, depart with their parents, or live out their short and very painful lives in a blaze of technological wizardry. The unit was immense, with space for over fifty tiny patients and the capacity to care for nearly two dozen ventilator-dependent children. On Wednesday, June 28, during work rounds on the first day of the rotation, I saw them all for the first time—infant after infant laid out on warming tables in nice straight rows, babies who looked barely human—and my anxiety and depression grew as we reviewed each new successive patient's history. By the end of rounds that morning, I seriously considered taking the elevator down to the ground floor of the hospital, walking out through the main entrance, getting into my car, and driving away, never to return. But I fought off the urge. To this day I'm still not exactly sure why.

I was assigned fourteen infants during work rounds my first morning. Five of my patients were relatively "fresh" preemies—recently born, critically ill babies who depended on the unit's ventilators to aid their premature lungs; three more were terminal cases who, because of the complications they'd suffered, had burned out both their lungs and their brains and therefore were left with no possible chance of surviving with any quality of life. Leaving work on Wednesday and Thursday evenings, I was extremely depressed. But that was nothing compared to the way I felt after completing my first night on call.

The night started off uneventfully. All the babies seemed more or less stable; besides, I was on call that night with Douglas Berkowitz, a very smart senior resident who knew a tremendous amount about neonatology. But my feelings of reassurance and calm were suddenly shattered at about nine o'clock when, while Doug and I were sitting in the staff lounge outside the NICU, our beepers simultaneously erupted. "Dr. Marion, report to the DR stat!" the box clipped to my belt ordered.

We were up and running within seconds. We pushed through the swinging doors of the delivery suite, located on the fourth floor one flight up from the NICU, just in time to come close to colliding with a gurney being pushed toward Delivery Room 3 at breakneck speed. The gurney, which bore a squirming woman, was being maneuvered by Tom Fredericks, and Al Schwartz, the obstetric residents on call that night. On seeing us, Fredericks shouted, "Crash section! Fetal distress—move it!"

Not comprehending precisely what was happening, I tailed Doug as, without a word, he headed into the locker room in the delivery suite. Following his lead, I pulled a fresh green scrub suit over my clothes and then rushed into DR 3, where the obstetric residents were already cutting skin.

Doug and I quickly prepared for the delivery of the infant. As ordered by the resident, I switched on the power supply of the warming table, the device on which the newborn would be laid after it was delivered, while Doug unwrapped two important bits of plastic tubing: one was an endotracheal tube that, if necessary, would be inserted down into the infant's trachea so that we could force oxygen directly into the lungs; the other bit of plastic was an umbilical artery line, a tube that could be inserted into one of the infant's umbilical arteries, allowing us to inject medications directly into the baby's bloodstream. After checking these tubes, the resident made sure that the medications we would need for emergency resuscitation, epinephrine, calcium, and bicarbonate, were all drawn up in syringes and ready for use. When he had determined that everything was in place, Doug handed me a sterile towel and told me to go catch the baby.

My knees shaking, I walked to the delivery table and waited. While the obstetricians worked, Tom Fredericks filled us in on the patient's history: "Three weeks postdate, from Nashua, New Hampshire," he said, concentrating most of his attention on the rapidly progressing surgery. "Transferred by ambulance. The damn thing broke down a few miles north of Boston. The trip took three hours. She ruptured membranes about an hour ago. Lots of meconium. She got here twenty minutes ago. We attached a monitor and got her ready. There was severe bradycardia with the last contraction, and the heart rate never came back up. So we called you guys and brought her back here."

What this meant was that the baby whose birth we were witnessing was in serious trouble. The bag of amniotic fluid which had surrounded the fetus had ruptured during the mother's ambulance ride to St. Anne's from New Hampshire, and rather than being clear, as amniotic fluid was supposed to be, the fluid that had gushed through the woman's birth canal during the ambulance ride had contained meconium, the greenish-brown substance of the fetus's first bowel movement. The presence of meconium in amniotic fluid is often a bad sign, implying that the fetus is, or has recently been, in physical distress. Low oxygen concentration in the baby's bloodstream often leads to the passage of meconium while the fetus is in the womb.

But besides being a signal that the fetus is in danger, the presence of meconium in the amniotic fluid itself poses a major problem: since the fetus must breathe soon after it departs the womb, any meconium that is in the infant's mouth will be aspirated, sucked deep down into the lungs. Such an occurrence frequently results in a condition known as meconium pneumonitis, a form of pneumonia which causes respiratory distress and a whole series of physiological disturbances that can prove life-threatening to the newborn.

Because of the meconium in the amniotic fluid the obstetric residents had attached to the mother the leads of a fetal heart monitor, a device that checks a baby's heart rate and responses to the normal stresses of labor. When the woman from New Hamsphire had had a contraction, the fetal monitor revealed a significant drop in the baby's heart rate. Often the heart rate of a fetus will return to normal after a contraction has ended; in this case, however, the heart rate remained at an abnormally low level, another sign that the child was in serious, perhaps worsening danger.

My knees continued to shake as I watched Fredericks and Schwartz perform the cesarean section. Their instruments moved rapidly, the reflection of the bright operating room lights off the surgical steel dazzling the eye. Less than six minutes after the surgeons had first cut through the skin of the woman's abdomen, the baby's head was visible, peaking through the incision. Seconds later, Tom Fredericks plopped the blood and meconium-splattered male infant onto the sterile towel I held out to him; running with the child toward the warming table, I saw that he was limp and appeared to be lifeless.

The baby was undoubtedly dead when he first reached the warming table. He was dead, and he would have been considered stillborn, but then Doug Berkowitz had gone to work. Wasting not a second, the resident was on the kid as soon as he hit the table. While I wiped the thick greenish fluid off the infant's lifeless body with the sterile towel, Doug, using a laryngoscope, an instrument designed to push away the tongue and shine a bright light into the back of the throat, attempted to pass the endotracheal tube through the baby's vocal cords and down into his windpipe. He got the thing in on his first attempt. Then, while securing the tube with tape, the resident instructed me to listen to the child's heart with my stethoscope and to beat out the rhythm I heard by tapping my index finger against one of the sides of the warming table.

Doing as I was told, I found that the heart rate at that point was about thirty, much lower than normal. While listening to the *tap tap tap* of my fingers, Doug, using a special catheter threaded through the endotracheal tube, suctioned out a large quantity of meconium which had passed into the baby's windpipe and lungs during the process of birth; after cleaning the trachea with a small amount of sterile water, he resuctioned, continuing the process until all traces of meconium were gone. The baby's heart rate was now down to twenty-five beats a minute; the infant was two minutes old.

Once he was sure that the airway was clear, the resident attached an ambu bag, a soft rubber balloon that continually refills itself with oxygen, to the end of the endotracheal tube and began pumping the gas into the baby's lungs at the rate of about forty puffs a minute. The baby responded almost immediately to the oxygen; his heart rate came up to sixty beats a minute. But it seemed stuck there, resistant to going any higher. Listening to the tapping of my index finger, Doug continued to pump on the ambu bag for another minute, but when the heart rate remained at sixty he decided it was time to try something else. The baby was now a little over three minutes old.

The resident ordered me to take over the management of the ambu bag. The nervousness I had been feeling intensified as I moved to the head of the warming table and took possession of the rubber bag, pumping on it just as Doug had done. Without hesitation, the resident grabbed a bottle of antiseptic solution and poured the sticky brown liquid over the lower half of the infant's abdomen. He then set about placing an umbilical artery catheter into the stump of the baby's umbilical cord.

Doug succeeded in getting the catheter into place on his second try. As I continued to pump on the ambu bag, the resident injected the syringes of medication through the umbilical artery line: first, bicarbonate, to counteract the effects of the lactic acid that had built up in the infant's blood as a result of his lack of oxygen; then epinephrine, to get the heart rate up into the normal range; and finally a solution of calcium. After the first round of medications had cleared the tubing and gotten into the baby's circulatory system, the resident pulled the earpieces of my stethoscope out of my ears, and placed them in his own. Closing his eyes, concentrating, he listened for the heart rate, tapping it out with his index finger against the wall of the warming table as I had done only minutes before. The baby's heart rate was now up to just over a hundred beats a minute. After two minutes of listening and beating his finger at a rock-steady rate—after convincing himself that the baby was now stable, ten minutes or so after he had been born—Doug said simply, "Let's get him out of here." We transferred the infant to the transport incubator, a Plexiglas box with wheels at the bottom and an oxygen supply at the head, and with Doug pushing and me still pumping on the ambu bag, we flew out of DR 3, out of the delivery suite, down the hall to the waiting elevator, and down to the third floor, where the NICU nurses had been preparing for our arrival. In all, about fifteen minutes had passed from the time our beepers went off to the time we returned, but it was the longest fifteen minutes of my life. And it was nothing compared to what was in store for us.

We were up all night with that baby. Although Doug Berkowitz had saved the kid's life in the delivery room, the infant, on his arrival in the NICU, was far from healthy, and it was touch and go with him for the remainder of the night. Because of the prenatal passage of meconium, and despite Doug's vigorous efforts to suction as much of the stuff out as he could, the baby developed severe pneumonia, his lungs becoming so stiff and sticky as a result of the meconium still trapped deep inside them that through the night it became necessary to use greater and greater amounts of pressure, generated by the mechanical ventilator to which we'd attached the baby on his arrival in the NICU, in order to force what was only a barely adequate amount of oxygen into the child's system. And the gradually increasing ventilator pressure itself led to additional problems nearly as life-threatening as the pneumonia itself: during the night the baby developed two separate pneumothoraces, episodes of collapsed lungs directly resulting from the high pressures we were using, complications that required the emergency placement of tubes plunged through the baby's chest wall and into his chest cavity in order to drain out the free air that had accumulated. But despite these complications, with Doug, one of the NICU nurses, and me by his side at all times, the baby survived the night.

It's amazing what a night without sleep, spent under intense, life-and-death pressure, can do to a human being. Sleep deprivation can take a reasonably well-balanced, relatively intact person and transform him into a maniac. And so, on the morning after my first on-call night spent without sleep, I had become uncontrollably emotionally unbalanced.

Terry Costa was more than a little surprised at the outburst that greeted her arrival that Saturday morning. The eruption of tears did nothing to relieve my sense of panic: my shortness of breath was becoming more critical, the hunger for air increasing with each passing minute. And so, quickly, I signed the NICU out to Terry, telling her only the barest of facts about the new baby as well as about what had happened to each of the other critically ill ventilator-dependent premature infants since she'd left for home the afternoon before. When I was done I fled from the hospital, my breathing becoming less labored the moment I hit the parking lot. And then I drove to the airport to pick up Beth.

This weekend was the first during which Beth took the Eastern shuttle from New York to Boston to visit me. During the months following Match Day, Beth and I had busied ourselves looking for suitable housing in the two cities, sorting out our belongings so we'd be sure to have what we needed where we needed it. As the late spring began to drift toward summer we had both begun to anticipate, if not actually look forward to, the challenges of life after medical school. "After all, how bad can it be?" we asked each other repeatedly.

In the middle of June, two weeks before my internship was scheduled to begin, we moved out of our apartment in the Bronx. Beth moved her clothes, books, and personal items into a tiny dormitory room on the campus at Columbia, while the remainder of the belongings we had accumulated during our one and a half years of marriage—furniture, dishes, and other possessions—were loaded onto a van and transported to the apartment we had rented in Watertown, a suburb about five miles west of Boston. Beth came up to help me unpack and get settled, and then, during the last week of June, she went back to New York to return to her lab work, leaving me alone in our apartment.

After a single day of orientation I had begun my internship on a Wednesday, three days before the morning I began to cry as Terry Costa congratulated me for having survived till the weekend. To my way of thinking, those three days were enough internship to last for the rest of my life.

I stopped the car at the curb outside the Eastern terminal at Logan Airport. The terminal entrance was unusually quiet; it was pretty early in the morning, and it seemed as if the airport was still asleep. I had gotten my emotions under control again; I hadn't shed a single tear since leaving St. Anne's, and I planned to keep it that way. So I sat, alone in the car, waiting for Beth's flight to arrive.

A rush of activity began within the confines of the building after about fifteen minutes. Most of them carrying small suitcases, people began briskly walking through the electric doors of the terminal and out into the already warm July morning. I stared at the exit door, searching the forms that came through, hunting for that familiar face. And then, all at once, there she was; I don't think I was ever so happy to see anyone before.

I got out of the car and walked toward Beth to greet her, falling into her arms just outside the passenger door. We embraced long and hard, and in total silence, and when that embrace ended we got into the car.

"How are you?" she asked. "I missed you so much."

I couldn't help it. I had no control over myself. Like a dam breaking, I burst into tears for the second time that morning. My wall of concentration had cracked into a million pieces; I sat behind the steering wheel of the car, crying, as I'd cried the year before in the emergency room at Jonas Bronck Hospital. I cried for those babies in the NICU at St. Anne's Hospital, the infants who, from the very beginning, had had little or no chance of surviving, who were being kept alive only because the technology needed to do so was available. I cried for the children's parents, who had been unfortunate enough to have given birth to infants who, in the best of worlds, would have been allowed to die peacefully, with dignity, and not forced to hang on and on, their inevitable deaths delayed for weeks and months by the machines of modern medicine. But the longest and loudest wail, the most sustained and gut-wrenching moan, the heaviest and hardest cry I cried was for me. Suddenly, for the first time since I had begun medical school four years before, I came to realize that this was not what I wanted out of life. I didn't want to spend every third night awake and at work; I had neither the strength nor the intelligence to manage such critically ill patients; I didn't have the willingness, the patience, or the perseverance to watch these children grow sicker and sicker, to watch them and their families suffer, to stand by doing nothing as they died and their parents mourned. In the front seat of our car that Saturday morning, as we sat motionless at the curb at the Eastern terminal, for the very first time in my life I felt trapped and deceived, trapped in a career for which I had never been prepared emotionally, caught in the reality when I'd only known the idealized version, deceived by a training system that had allowed this to take place.

So began Beth's first weekend in Boston. In the years we've spent together since, through the good times and the bad, we've never once discussed that weekend in early July. I don't know for sure exactly what was running through Beth's mind during that Saturday morning as she listened to me cry. She had to figure that something terrible had happened to me, that the people who ran that residency program had taken her husband and altered his mind, that for the rest of her married life, or at least until I finished my training, she would be forced to spend her time with a man she'd once loved but who, through some horrible twist in the path leading from medical student to practicing physician, had been transformed into a maniac. But on that Saturday morning, in the front seat of the car, Beth didn't reveal any of these thoughts to me; instead she sat by, quietly supportive. In doing so, she probably saved my professional life.

Beth put her arms around me; she hugged me, comforted me, let me cry on her shoulder. We sat like that, outside the terminal building, for nearly an hour. The hustle and bustle of the day now coming to life at the airport went on all around us as we sat locked in an embrace, silent except for the sound of my crying.

When I at last recovered some semblance of control, Beth moved me into the passenger seat, took her place behind the wheel, and drove the car out of the airport. The silence in the car continued during the trip home to Watertown. In the parking lot outside our apartment, Beth helped me out of the car, took me upstairs, and put me to bed. I fell asleep almost immediately and slept soundly until six o'clock that evening.

I felt better after I woke up, and my emotions were more under control. We went out for dinner, then back to bed. By Sunday morning I was relaxed and nearly recovered. By Monday I was ready to face the preemies of the St. Anne's NICU one more time.

That's pretty much how the first month of my internship went, bringing on chronic depression without interruption. Almost continually that month I felt powerless, frustrated, and trapped. By the end of July I had had all I could take of the NICU at St. Anne's Hospital. What I desperately wanted was to get back to our main hospital, the Boston Medical Center, and spend time in more normal pediatric service. But by a stroke of horrible luck, I wound up spending August as well in an intensive care unit. The neonatal intensive care unit back at the Boston Medical Center was much smaller and not nearly as intimidating as the unit at St. Anne's. But the size didn't make that much difference, at least not to me.

8

Starting an IV

**Second month of internship,
August 1978**

A drop of sweat fell from my forehead as I pushed the
tiny needle through the skin of M/C (short for Male
Child) O'Hara's right hand. Barbara, one of the night
nurses in the neonatal intensive care unit at the Boston
Medical Center, leaned over the infant, holding his
wasted arm steady, trying to prevent the child from pulling away or jerking in response to the sensation of pain
the penetration of the needle would almost certainly pro-
duce. But as far as I could tell there wasn't any need for
Barbara to hold the kid so tightly: there wasn't much
chance that M/C O'Hara would pull away or jerk or make
any other kind of spontaneous movement on his own,
either now or at any time in the future. The portions of
his brain responsible for controlling the movement of his
muscles, like most of the rest of the infant's central nervous system, had been too severely damaged to respond
to pain, or any other kind of external stimulation.

M/C O'Hara, who was just over three months old, had
weighed less than a pound and a half at birth. Born more
than fourteen weeks premature, he had nearly died in the
delivery room at South Shore Community Hospital.
Looking back, it probably would have been better for
everyone involved if his death had been allowed to occur.

but instead he'd received heroic care from the neonatologist who was called in, and the superhuman effort put forth by that physician succeeded in saving the child. After being stabilized at South Shore, M/C O'Hara was transported up to Boston Medical Center by ambulance, and within two hours of his birth he was plugged in to the vast technological dynamo that was the NICU, where machines of all types had been programmed to keep him breathing and keep his heart beating.

During his first weeks in the NICU, while M/C O'Hara lay critically ill, everything imaginable was done to keep him going. He spent his entire first month of life attached by tubing to a mechanical ventilator, a machine that pumped oxygen into his immature lungs forty times a minute. Incapable of either sucking or swallowing on his own, initially because of prematurity but ultimately owing to brain damage, for his first two months he was fed formula introduced through a tube that had been passed through his nose and into his stomach. But then, at two months, because of an inflammation of the intestine—a condition known as necrotizing enterocolitis, which caused his abdomen to become distended and his stools discolored by blood—even these tube feedings had to be discontinued. The infant had since received all his nutrition by vein in the form of an intravenous solution called "total parenteral nutrition," or TPN. All during this time M/C O'Hara's heart rate, breathing rate, blood pressure, and temperature were checked continuously by our state-of-the-art electronic monitoring equipment, and loud alarms sounded every time a perturbation in any of these vital signs was registered by one of the machines. With all the tubes going in and the monitor leads coming out, it was difficult to tell exactly where M/C O'Hara ended and the technology began.

But other than keeping the unfortunate infant alive, this vigorous care had done M/C O'Hara little good. By the time he was a month old it had become clear to everyone that, because of lack of oxygen during the first few hours of life, the infant's brain was badly damaged, a condition technically known as hypoxic-ischemic encephalopathy. When I first met him early in August, the baby was a virtual vegetable; unable to interact with anything or anyone in his environment, dependent on artificial treatments in order to maintain his basic life functions, abandoned by his parents who, after weeks of worsening reports about their firstborn child's medical condition, finally came to understand the full implications of his prematurity, M/C O'Hara was little more than a human pincushion, a tiny object with essentially no prognosis and almost no remaining usable veins. Since the infant relied exclusively on intravenous feedings for his survival, and since the attending physician in charge of the NICU that month had decided, for reasons that were not completely clear to me, that the child would survive, this latter fact meant nothing but trouble to me and the other interns assigned to work in the unit.

I was only eight weeks into my internship that night, and I was feeling pretty frustrated. I had come to Boston at the end of June with, I thought, a reasonably good attitude: I had wanted to do a good job during internship, to take excellent care of the patients who were assigned to me, to offer comfort and support to their parents, and to learn everything I needed to know in order to become an outstanding pediatrician. I had understood that I would need to work hard to achieve these goals—all new interns realize that they are going to lose a lot of sleep, spending long days in the hospital in order to learn the craft of medicine; but I'd thought I wouldn't mind the long hours and the lack of sleep if at the end I would achieve my objective.

Then I began my internship year in the neonatal intensive care unit at St. Anne's Hospital, and I developed second thoughts. Many of the patients I cared for at St. Anne's were critically ill, hanging on to life by little more than a prayer and some tubing that connected them to the port of a ventilator. The place was filled with the sadness of broken hopes and shattered lives, and I came away from the experience more depressed than I ever imagined would be possible while working in the field of pediatrics.

I made it through my rotation at St. Anne's only to find, on my return to the Boston Medical Center, where I would spend the remainder of my internship, that I had been scheduled to work for a second consecutive month in a NICU. When I learned of this apparent scheduling screw-up I rushed to the chief resident's office, complaining loudly and vehemently about this horrible injustice. The chief, who was responsible for making up the schedule, responded to my complaint with little sympathy. "Sorry, but there's nothing I can do about it," he told me. "It's too late to change it now. I'll try to make it up to you later in the year. In the meantime, just hang in there." And I did try to hang in there but, by the last week of August, as I stood poised over M/C O'Hara with that needle held firmly in my hand, I'd just about reached the end of my rope.

Starting intravenous lines in M/C O'Hara had become pure torture. Every day, it seemed, he needed to have a new line started because, owing to the fragility of his blood vessels, the one that had been placed only the day before would invariably become infiltrated, spilling irritating TPN solution into the soft tissues of his arm or leg. Each of us interns spent hour after hour during our nights on call trying to locate yet another vein that might hold a needle. We searched and poked and prodded, constantly cursing at this tiny, inanimate child. In the process of restarting his IV, we would lose any possibility of getting some sleep.

That night, however, I had been lulled into a false sense of complacency. The senior resident had started a new intravenous line in the baby late that afternoon, and I allowed myself to believe that I would be safe at least until the next morning. But then, at around two-thirty in the morning—just as I was finishing the chores on the list of scut work which had been signed out to me by the two other interns before they left for home at a little after

six o'clock and I was beginning to imagine what the
sheets of the bed in the on-call room would feel like
against the skin of my legs—the page I'd been dreading
came. "O'Hara's IV's out," Barbara said when I answered. "Can you come by and put in a new one?"

So Barbara and I now stood over M/C O'Hara, who
was lying motionless on the warming table in the treatment room directly across the hall from the neonatal intensive care unit. The room, which was nothing more
than a supply closet that had been converted into a place
for performing invasive procedures on NICU patients,
was steaming hot. Although it was nearly three o'clock
in the morning, we were in the midst of a heat wave and
the temperature in downtown Boston just then was easily
over ninety degrees. The treatment room, along with the
rest of the pediatric wing of the Boston Medical Center,
had not been blessed with central air conditioning; by
the time I gathered up all the supplies I would need to
start the IV, collecting alcohol swabs, sterile gauze pads,
a syringe filled with saline solution, a supply of rubber
bands to be used as tourniquets, and a jumbo box of tiny
preemie-sized butterfly needles, the fresh green scrub suit
into which I'd changed just after midnight was completely soaked with sweat.

As expected, the baby failed to move even an inch as
the needle I wielded pierced his flesh. Without hesitation
I began angling the needle's tip upward, toward what,
using my vivid imagination, I believed might be a blood
vessel—nothing more really, than a tiny blue line just
barely visible through the skin. Slowly, with great care,
I directed the needle forward until its hub lay flush against
the baby's skin; but no blood appeared in the tubing. "I
must have missed it," I mumbled. Barbara nodded.
Gently, I pulled the needle back so that, as before, only
the tip lay under the skin; then again, slowly and delib-
erately, I advanced the needle forward. But once more,
when the needle hub hit skin no blood appeared. "I'm
almost positive there's something there," I said, gazing
up almost pleadingly at the nurse. "The vein must be

moving around.'' I began to pull back on the needle a second time, but when it was about halfway out, blood suddenly started to fill the tubing. ''Damn!'' I shouted. ''I hit it on the way out! It never works when you hit the vein on the way out.''

''Are you sure?'' Barbara asked. ''It looks pretty good to me. Why don't you try hooking up the IV solution and see what happens?''

''I'm sure it's going to infiltrate,'' I replied, but I did as the nurse suggested anyway. I hooked up the tubing coming from the bag of IV solution which hung suspended from a steel hook in the treatment room ceiling and slowly opened the control valve. While watching the flow I wiped the sweat from my forehead and cheeks with a paper towel. Within a minute, an egg-shaped swelling appeared under the skin around the site of the needle. The vein had infiltrated.

I sighed, pulled the needle out of the baby's hand, and jabbed it angrily into the mattress of the warming table. ''Where are you going to try next?'' the nurse asked.

''I think there might be something up in the left elbow.'' I moved toward the baby's left arm and took a second butterfly needle from its sterile package.

''That's where his last IV was,'' Barbara said, stepping into the place I had just vacated. ''That vein's already been blown.''

''I'll try to snake the needle in above the infiltrate,'' I replied, wrapping the rubber band tourniquet around the infant's left upper arm and beginning to search the elbow. There was a big vein there all right, and I was sure I'd be able to get a needle into it without any problem, but the area did look red and raw, the result, as Barbara had pointed out, of the previously infiltrated IV. But hell, red and raw or not, a vein's a vein! I gingerly passed the tip of the new needle through the skin above the elbow, just to the side of where the big vein bulged. Once again, after the baby failed to move even an inch when the needle entered his skin, I slowly advanced it until blood began to fill its hub.

"Great," I said, nodding my head, "that one felt good." Pulling off the tourniquet, again allowing myself to imagine the feel of sheets against my skin, I continued: "Now we'll just hook up the tubing, cover the whole thing with tape, and Mr. O'Hara will be back in business."

Barbara hooked up the IV solution tubing and opened the valve while, my mind now at ease, I began the intricate job of taping this obviously excellent new IV in place. I had used up a huge wad of tape when the nurse next spoke: "Bob, I don't like the look of that elbow."

I hesitated a few seconds, looking up at her with anger in my eyes. "We don't have to like the way it looks, Barbara," I finally replied, going back to completing my taping job. "All we have to worry about is that the damned thing's running."

"But I think it's infiltrated," the nurse said. "It looks like it's starting to blow up."

I took a long look at the elbow. It did look puffy, but hell, that could easily have been the result of the previous IV. "And the drip's not running all that well," the nurse added. I looked at the drip chamber attached to the bag of IV solution; a drop would fall, then nothing would happen for five or six seconds; then another drop would fall.

"Damn!" I groaned, at last convinced that this IV too wasn't going to work. I began ripping off all the tape I'd placed so artistically and pulled out the needle. "Can't we get any more air in here?" I yelled as I jabbed the needle into the mattress, next to the last one. The treatment room didn't have any windows, and its only door was already wide open.

"Why don't we take a little break and cool off?" the nurse asked.

"No," I snapped while wrapping the rubber band tourniquet around the baby's left leg. "I just want to get this damned thing over with."

I searched that leg and foot for nearly five minutes but didn't find a single vein anywhere. Sweat had fallen into

my eyes; they were now burning, and my vision began
to get blurry. I pulled the rubber band off the left leg and
wrapped it tight around the right. I inspected that leg and
foot also, holding the skin very close to my eyes, but
again I could find nothing. "I'm going to have to try for
the head," I finally said, reaching for one of the surgical
prep sets that were stored on a shelf in the treatment
room. Putting intravenous lines into the veins of the
scalp, although somewhat gruesome when described, is
a completely acceptable treatment in newborns. And so,
after tearing the set open and taking out the disposable
razor inside, I began to shave some of the thin hair from
the left side of the baby's scalp. "Look at that!" I said
when I'd cleared most of the hair. "A pipeline!"

"I think that might be the temporal artery, Bob," Barbara said, but I wouldn't listen. I knew you weren't supposed to start an IV in an artery, that such an action
might be fraught with complications, but I didn't care; I
just wanted to be finished and get to bed. So I pulled a
rubber band over the baby's scalp and, with a new needle
in hand, went for the vessel. Bright red blood began to
fill the hub of the needle almost as soon as I got it under
the skin; I cut the rubber band tourniquet with the razor,
hooked up the bag of IV solution, and slowly opened the
valve.

As the fluid went through the needle, the skin of the
baby's scalp began to blanch. The blanching rapidly
spread until a three-inch circle of skin had turned sick-
eningly white. "Damn!" I shouted, realizing that I had
in fact stuck the needle into the baby's temporal artery.
I began banging my fist against the table on which I had
laid out all the supplies.

"Be careful when you take that out!" Barbara ordered,
now losing patience with me. I did as she said, again
angrily stabbing the used needle into the mattress.

"Maybe you should let the resident give it a try," Barbara suggested, but I didn't respond. I was too frustrated
to stop now: I had to start this IV myself. I tied a new
rubber band around the baby's left leg, carefully search-

ing the area a second time, but again, no vein was visible. That's when I decided to try a blind stick. From the anatomy course I'd taken in the first year of medical school, I remembered the exact location of the long saphenous vein as it coursed its way upward from the foot. Unwrapping yet another needle, I jabbed its tip under the skin right near the inner malleolus, the bone that forms the bump on the inside of the ankle, and rapidly advanced the needle forward. Nothing happened. I pulled the needle back and rammed it forward again. Still no blood appeared. I tried a third time, and then a fourth, and then a fifth, just jabbing that needle forward and pulling it back, again and again. Never did any blood enter the tubing; never was a functioning intravenous line established. Barbara stood by watching me, horrified as I jabbed the baby's leg over and over again, until at last she commanded, "Bob, enough is enough! Take out that needle right now, and call the resident!"

I stopped and stared at her; my eyes were burning, my scrub suit was soaked, and the insides of my sneakers were damp with perspiration. I had been working without a break in the NICU for nineteen straight hours, handling one emergency after the next, restarting IVs, trying to track down X rays that had evidently been irretrievably lost; I'd argued with laboratory technicians who refused to perform tests on such small quantities of blood, and with the neonatal attending who didn't seem to want to listen to reason. I was tired and frustrated and angry— angry at the nurse for ordering me around, angry at the hospital for not being air-conditioned, angry at the weather bureau, which I figured should be held responsible for the heat wave, angry at my medical school adviser for even suggesting that I look into the residency program of the Boston Medical Center when I was applying for internships the year before, angry at this baby, who, in addition to everything else that was wrong with him, apparently didn't possess a single, solitary, visible vein within the confines of his entire body which would successfully hold a tiny butterfly needle. But most of all

I was angry at myself for failing, angry because I couldn't get a simple IV started.

I must have stood there, transfixed, staring at Barbara for more than a minute. When the trance was finally broken I took a deep breath, pulled the needle out of the baby's foot, and stabbed it into the mattress next to the others. Then, still fuming, I walked off to the nurses' station and dialed the number of the senior resident's on-call room.

That scene in the treatment room of the neonatal intensive care unit at the Boston Medical Center occurred only nineteen months after the early morning during my third-year clerkship in internal medicine when I'd stood and watched as my intern, Al Barrister, had nearly exploded simply because our patient Mrs. Schwab, had committed the sin of staying alive too long. Her spiking a fever had forced Al into having to draw her blood, thus depriving him of the chance of getting a few hours' sleep. It was only a little more than a year and a half since I'd promised myself that I would never, ever allow myself to think about a patient the way Al Barrister had thought about poor Mrs. Schwab, but here I was, only eight weeks into my internship, sadistically stabbing needles into the skin of a severely damaged infant whose only crime was that he had run out of usable veins.

The truth of the matter was that I had come to hate this patient—an eventuality that, just two years before, had never even occurred to me as a remote possibility. But here I was, less than two months into my internship, as exhausted, as angry, and as depressed as Al Barrister had been during the month I'd worked with him. My God, if this had happened to me in August, what was I going to be like in February?

But life improved. August ended, and I moved out of the NICU, never—as the chief resident promised—to return, at least not during the remainder of my internship. My next few rotations weren't as stressful: I spent September working on the general pediatric floor and October on the infectious disease floor. But though life seemed better, when I compared my existence during internship with the life I'd led during medical school, I realized something was missing, some intangible that I couldn't quite identify was absent from my life. It would take until January for me to figure out this mystery.

In November, I did the first of my three scheduled rotations in the outpatient department. My duties during that month proved to be a great relief: the days I spent in the emergency room and pediatric clinics were the first during my internship when I actually enjoyed my work. At least I enjoyed it until I came down with a bad case of the flu near the end of the month.

9

Giving Directions

**Fifth month of internship,
November 1978**

I was in trouble. It was late November, we were in the
middle of an outbreak of the flu, and by five o'clock that
afternoon, the time I began my overnight shift, the waiting area of the pediatric emergency room was filled with
children of all ages who were febrile, sore, stuffed up,
sneezing, and basically feeling horrible. To make matters
worse, I had begun to feel sick myself the night before,
my head slightly achy and my throat sort of scratchy, and
I had awakened that morning in a cold sweat, feeling
miserable; I was barely able to hold my head erect on
my shoulders. The forces against which I'd been battling
had won the war: I'd developed a whopping case of the
flu. Rather than staying awake all night here in the emergency room, caring for patients, most of whom would
probably turn out to be far less sick than I was, the thing
I really wanted to do was walk down the hall to the pediatric on-call room, lie down on the cot, and die as
quickly and as quietly as possible. But I knew that this
wish would not be granted; I was, after all, an intern,
and interns are supposed to work, even when they're sick.

So, after squeaking a hoarse hello to the head nurse
and unpacking my stethoscope and other equipment in
one of the examining rooms, I prepared to begin my

work: I opened a box of hospital-grade facial tissues, the special "extra scratchy" variety so popular at medical centers, cracked open a fresh bottle of Dimetapp decongestant, and after taking a swig, slowly began making my way through the pile of charts that had been laid out for me by the triage nurse. As I set about my work, I prayed that no very sick children were lurking in there among all those coughing, sneezing, crying wretches.

Every one of the patients seemed to have the same set of symptoms, a fact that made my work much easier. By the fourth patient I had gotten down a fairly comfortable routine: I would listen intently for two entire minutes as one of the child's parents related the history; then I'd spend about three minutes performing a physical examination, the sole purpose of which was to confirm in my own mind that the kid didn't have anything really serious; then, as the parents busied themselves with putting the kid's clothes back on, I'd talk for a minute or two about the natural history of this particular strain of the influenza virus, telling the parents that the illness seemed to be taking approximately five days to run its course; and finally, after answering their questions, I'd send them on their way, back to their homes, with strict instructions to keep the kid in bed, give him plenty of liquids to drink, and have him take Tylenol every four hours. (These instructions had not been learned during my four years of medical school, nor had I figured them out during the first four and a half months of my internship; rather, I had picked up this important medical advice from the thousands of hours I'd spent watching television commercials throughout my life.) If I threw in a couple of minutes to fill out the chart, blow my nose, complain to the nurses about how rotten I was feeling, and maybe take another dose of Tylenol or Dimetapp, I found I was able to complete a patient visit, from greeting to farewell, in just under thirteen minutes.

At about six-thirty, as I was making my way through my seventh patient's history, I heard my name called over the loudspeaker. It was the triage nurse, ordering me out into the waiting area, stat. Leaving my patient and her mother in mid-sentence, I rushed out to the waiting room, expecting to find some horrible medical disaster awaiting me. Instead, however, I found the triage nurse pointing upward toward one of the room's walls.

Mounted on the wall was a television set, and on the screen I recognized the long, thin face of Dr. Oscar Bloomenfeld, world-famous clinical geneticist, professor of pediatrics at the Boston Medical Center, and medical correspondent for one of the local television stations. Standing next to Dr. Bloomenfeld was Dr. Ralph Simpson, director of the infectious disease service at our hospital. Inching closer to the set, I recognized the location: the two physicians were standing in the hallway outside the infectious disease ward of the pediatric wing. And after listening for just a few seconds, I realized with a sinking feeling that Dr. Bloomenfeld was interviewing Dr. Simpson about the epidemic of Kawasaki disease that had recently hit the Boston area.

Over the previous few weeks, all of us interns and residents had learned far more about the mysterious disorder called Kawasaki disease than any of us ever wanted to know. The epidemic started unassumingly enough in early October, when a fifteen-month-old boy from Waltham, a suburb northwest of Boston, was admitted to the infectious disease ward for evaluation. For nearly a week prior to his admission, the child had been running an extremely high fever and had had a painful red throat, markedly swollen lymph nodes in his neck, and a bright red rash on his skin which extended from his head to his toes. In the hospital he remained burning hot, with temperatures ranging between 104 and 106 degrees for over a week. Despite our best efforts and a million-dollar workup, no obvious infectious source causing these symptoms could be identified. Finally, on the eighth day of hospitalization, when the child's fever finally broke, dropping into the normal range for the first time in nearly two weeks, the superficial layer of skin around the boy's fingernails began to peel off in long strips. This bizarre phenomenon confirmed the diagnosis Dr. Simpson had been entertaining since the boy was first admitted: the child had Kawasaki disease.

Kawasaki disease was a relatively new disorder then, having first been reported in the early seventies. Since all the initial cases had occurred in Japan, the disease was for some time believed to be a geographically isolated entity, a peculiar syndrome limited in its distribution to the Far East. But then, in 1974, a smattering of cases were first recognized within the continental United States. Dr. Simpson, who in the past few years had diagnosed and treated a handful of patients with Kawasaki disease at our medical center, at first believed that the case of the boy from Waltham was like all the others he'd seen: an isolated phenomenon, this single patient had mysteriously popped up for reasons no one could adequately explain.

But Dr. Simpson was wrong. Within a week of the time the boy was diagnosed, three other children from the western suburbs of Boston were admitted to our hospital with high fevers; these children also ultimately showed all the classic symptoms of Kawasaki disease. The next week brought a half-dozen more cases, and by the middle of November nearly half the beds on the infectious disease ward were filled with patients in the acute phase of Kawasaki disease. All of them were febrile, swollen, and incredibly irritable; these children could do little more than lie in their cribs, and in unison, constantly emit a high-pitched, irritating screech. We were clearly in the midst of an unprecedented epidemic of this unusual disorder, a cluster of patients larger than any ever seen outside Japan. And that night, seemingly at the very height of the epidemic, Dr. Simpson decided to go public with this information. So, forgetting for a minute the long backup of flu patients waiting to be seen, I stood and watched the interview as it played out on the television screen in the waiting area.

* * *

"It starts out looking something like a strep throat," Dr. Simpson was saying in his high-pitched nasal twang. "The children have high fever that lasts for at least five days, sore throats with redness of the mucous membranes, swollen, cracked lips, enlarged lymph nodes, or swollen glands as they're usually called, in the region of the neck, conjunctivitis, or pink eye, skin rashes, and swelling of the hands and feet. Eventually, after about a week or so, the fever drops and the skin around the fingernails begins to peel."

Oscar Bloomenfeld, who had been listening to Dr. Simpson's monologue intently, occasionally nodding his head to emphasize to the audience that he hadn't yet fallen into a deep sleep, finally asked, "Are there any long-term dangers associated with Kawasaki disease?"

"Oh, yes," the infectious disease expert replied without hesitation. "A small but significant percentage of children affected with the early symptoms of Kawasaki disease will go on to develop aneurysms, or swellings, of the coronary arteries, the vessels that carry blood and oxygen to the muscle of the heart. As a result of these aneurysms, some children with Kawasaki disease will go on to suffer heart attacks, or will even die suddenly, without any warning."

"Heart attacks and sudden death," Dr. Bloomenfeld repeated somberly. "Dr. Simpson, it sounds to me as if it would be very important for parents who think that their child has the symptoms of Kawasaki disease to have that child carefully checked out by a doctor."

"Very important," Dr. Simpson agreed, matching Dr. Bloomenfeld's funereal tone. And then, with his face turned directly toward the camera, Dr. Simpson uttered these fateful words: "If you suspect that your child has Kawasaki disease, contact your doctor immediately, or bring him to the pediatric emergency room at the Boston Medical Center." And, as my mouth dropped open, the telephone number of the ER was flashed across the screen.

* * *

"Oh, no!" I groaned. On this of all nights, when I was sick myself and the emergency room was already packed, the director of the infectious disease service had to get on the evening news and tell all the parents of Boston that if their kid had a fever and a sore throat they'd better get over to my emergency room or else the kid might have a heart attack and die. That night nearly every kid in Boston had a fever and a sore throat, but they sure as hell didn't all have Kawasaki disease; they had the damned flu!

The phones started ringing almost immediately; the lines were lighting up like a Christmas tree. My progress through the ever-growing pile of charts of patients waiting to be seen was all but halted as I was soon swamped trying to handle the calls from parents who didn't want their kids to fall over suddenly and die. Most of the calls were legitimate, concerning children with fever and other symptoms that overlapped with those Dr. Simpson had reported as occurring in Kawasaki disease. Some I was able to dismiss out of hand as nothing more than a mild case of the flu. Many, however, I couldn't be sure about over the phone, so I instructed the parents to bundle their kids up and bring them into the emergency room as soon as possible, wasting even more time as I gave careful directions about how to get to our medical center from Watertown, Waltham, or one of the other outlying suburbs.

But some of the calls I received that night were ridiculous, providing ample evidence that the Boston metropolitan area had at least as many loonies per capita as any other major city in the United States. One woman called to tell me that twelve years before her son, who had then been one and a half, had had a high fever, skin rash, enlarged lymph nodes, and swelling of his hands and feet, the exact symptoms of Kawasaki disease; but rather than diagnosing Kawasaki disease, the doctors who evaluated the kid made a diagnosis of leukemia. Although her son had received five years' worth of aggressive chemotherapy and made a complete recovery, the mother was now calling because she wanted me to make a retrospective, over-the-phone diagnosis of Kawasaki disease, thus freeing the boy from the "stigma of cancer" which still haunted him. Another woman stated that although her six-month-old daughter hadn't recently had a fever or rash, she had been drooling a lot more than usual, and the mother wanted to make sure that excessive salivation wasn't a symptom of Kawasaki disease which Dr. Simpson had neglected to mention during his appearance on the news. "No," I told her, "it sounds to me as if your daughter might just be teething."

"Yeah, that's what I thought," the woman replied. "I just wanted to make sure."

On and on into the night it went, the calls continuing to come from all over the Boston area, and all the children with the flu whose parents didn't want them to die suddenly of a heart attack continuing to register at the front desk. And even though I was popping Tylenol every four hours and drinking ounce after ounce of my decongestant elixir, I felt sicker and sicker as the night wore on, and I seriously doubted that I'd ever make it through to see the morning light. "Please, God," I prayed, "make all this stop."

But my prayers went unanswered; in fact, at least for a while, things seemed to get a lot worse. As if it hadn't caused enough trouble the first time it had been shown, Oscar Bloomenfeld's interview with Dr. Simpson was repeated on the local station's eleven o'clock news broadcast, which set off a new barrage of business. At about eleven-thirty I took a call from a man in Watertown who, after watching the news, had decided to check with me because his two-year-old son had many of the symptoms Dr. Simpson had mentioned. After listening to the story and realizing that the child sounded genuinely sick, and that the diagnosis could not be determined over the phone, I advised the man to bring his son in. "How do I get to your hospital, Doctor?" the man asked.

All at once the answer to my prayers came to me.

Without hesitation I asked, "Do you know where Long-wood Avenue is?"

"Sure," the man replied.

"Great. The address is three hundred Longwood Avenue. The sign outside says Boston Children's Hospital. Just go into the emergency room entrance and tell the nurse that you're concerned that your child might have Kawasaki disease. She'll take care of you right away."

"Thanks a lot, Doc," the man replied gratefully. "We'll be right over."

The solution seemed brilliant. Why should I, in my infirm state, spend the rest of the night killing myself? I had found an unbeatable secret weapon: I simply sent anyone who called and asked for directions over to Children's, the other major pediatric facility in Boston.

My plan worked perfectly. Although the calls kept coming, the siege of registering patients stopped abruptly at a little after midnight. By three o'clock, exhausted, overdosed on analgesics and decongestants, having killed off two whole boxes of tissues, and more than ready to curl up and die, I had seen them all; I retired to the on-call room a happy man and, undisturbed, slept soundly until seven-thirty the next morning.

In order to survive an internship, young doctors, whose lives rarely follow a straight and narrow path, finally need to take themselves in hand and feel confident enough to give directions. Sometimes, the best directions are the ones that lead to another hospital.

The epidemic of Kawasaki disease which gripped Boston during that late fall and early winter continued for a little over two months. During that period more than sixty children were diagnosed with the condition, making it the largest single outbreak of the syndrome ever to occur within the United States up to that time. I had the opportunity to take care of a good many of those sixty patients because after my rotation in the emergency room ended one week after that night, I moved on to a month-long assignment on the infectious disease ward.

Caring for these patients wasn't easy. The children felt miserable, and worse, each could potentially develop life-threatening complications. Our days at work and our nights on call were filled with many unpleasant tasks, including ordering electrocardiograms, echocardiograms, and other tests to monitor the functioning of the patients' hearts; drawing sample after sample of blood, attempting to identify the underlying cause of this weird disorder; trying our best to reassure the frightened parents that the odds were that everything would turn out all right and their children would be fine; and most difficult of all, listening for hours as the patients in the ward cried in a grating, high-pitched whine.

Over 50 percent of the children who were hospitalized during the epidemic suffered some type of complication involving their hearts. Many of the kids had aneurysms of the coronary arteries which ultimately resolved, but two of our patients, right before our eyes, had heart attacks during their stay in the hospital. Both of these children survived, but standing by their cribs, watching as their chest pain developed and worsened, documenting the characteristic electrocardiographic changes as they took place, and knowing that nothing any of us could do would make any difference, was one of the most frustrating and helpless feelings I'd ever had.

And then, just as suddenly as it had come, the epidemic ended. By the beginning of January no new cases of Kawasaki disease were being identified anywhere in New England. Why the initial outbreak occurred and what ultimately caused it to subside remains a mystery.

That November marked the high point of my internship. After a rough and terrifying start of the year, I was finally enjoying the work I was doing; there were even some mornings I genuinely didn't mind getting out of bed in order to come to the hospital. And it was in November that Beth decided to take a leave of absence from

10

The Morning After

It had been a long night, and I badly needed to get some
sleep. Beginning the previous afternoon and continuing
through the night and into the early morning hours, I'd
admitted patient after patient to the general pediatrics
ward. I had no idea what had caused so many seriously
ill children, each with out-of-control diabetes, a difficult
to treat form of cancer, or some other complicated medical condition, to require hospitalization for evaluation
and treatment during this one short span of eighteen
hours, but it happened. With the paranoia that had begun
to dominate my thinking, I had come to the conclusion
that it must all have stemmed from the fact that someone
was out to get me.

Someone *was* out to get me, I was sure, and I understood that it was now only a matter of time, but regardless of the cause of my bad luck during that night on call,
all of these patients had arrived, and all of them needed
immediate attention. And so, through the night, without
a moment's rest, without the opportunity to eat dinner or
breakfast, or to call my wife, or even to go to the bathroom, I had stayed awake, working my ass off, spending
the hours running from one disaster to the next, writing
admission notes and orders for the nurses, drawing blood

from and starting intravenous lines in veins scarred and irreparably damaged by years of treatment with sclerosing chemotherapeutic agents, performing difficult spinal taps on children who were, to say the least, not exactly cooperative, who kicked and punched and bit and spat each time I went anywhere near them with a needle. I had spent the night and early morning haunting the clinical laboratories and the nurses' station and treatment room in the general pediatric ward, performing electrocardiograms, ordering stat X rays and CAT scans and echocardiograms; I had called and awakened attending physicians from subspecialty consult services who were less than ecstatic to hear my voice on the other end of the phone in the middle of the night, but from whom I'd urgently needed advice regarding the management of one or another of the ward's new patients. It had been brutal, and for a time I thought it would be impossible to get through it, but somehow I had survived: I'd made it through to see the light of day. Now it was morning and the relief, the rest of our ward team, had arrived to rescue me.

By the time the siege ended I had admitted a total of sixteen patients, five of whom had been sick enough to qualify for admission to the pediatric intensive care unit. During work rounds the next morning I was so sleepy and overwhelmed that I had trouble remembering even the names of all of the new patients and their primary diagnoses; no way could I recall the finer details of their past histories, or of the recent medical problems that had prompted their physicians to send them to the hospital for admission. As Ted Young, the senior resident in charge of the ward that month, led Andrea Mishkin and Cindy Morris, the two other interns on our team, and me down the main corridor of the ward on work rounds, reviewing everything that had happened to each of the patients the previous night, it was clear to everyone that relying on me for information that morning was hopeless. "You're a wreck," Ted said before we'd even made it a third of the way through rounds. "Your being here isn't doing any of us any good. Why don't you go down to the on-call room and get some sleep before attending rounds start?''

"But I've got to tell you about the rest of last night's admissions," I replied halfheartedly. "And I've got all this scut work to do. I can't just go off and leave it."

"We'll figure out who's new and who was here yesterday," Ted replied. "And the other interns and I will pitch in and get your scut work done. Don't worry about it. Just give us your notes from last night and get lost."

The senior resident didn't need to make the offer twice: I knew a couple hours' sleep wasn't going to cure everything that was wrong with me that morning, but I also knew it wouldn't hurt, either. And so, without another word of protest, I walked off the ward in the direction of the converted laundry closet that, during an uncharacteristic moment of blind generosity some years before, the medical center's administrators had set aside as an on-call room for the pediatric interns and residents.

At last off-duty and at ease, I happily entered the on-call room. Furnished with an old set of battered bunk beds, a telephone stand, and the room's single most important element, a telephone, it had no radiator or window, making it unbearably hot in the summer and icy cold in the winter. It was rarely adequately cleaned, and despite the passage of time, it still reeked of the dirty laundry that had been stored in it years before. But on that particular morning, following the night I'd just had, that tiny room seemed almost like heaven. I removed my sneakers, socks, and tie almost ecstatically, then climbed up the ladder into the top bunk, the bed in which, had things gone a little better, I would have spent at least a couple of hours the night before. As my worries dropped away and I rapidly began to enter Dreamland, out of the clear blue, in a shriek of high-pitched, irritating noise, my beeper suddenly exploded.

"Son of a bitch!" I yelled, instantly hurtled back into consciousness. Carefully stepping down the ladder, making sure not to miss a wrung, I stiffly reached across the lower bunk to the telephone stand. Dialing the all-too-familiar number of the page operator, nearly blind with a combination of anger at this disturbance and exhaustion, I growled to myself, "This better be damned important!"

The phone rang seven times before someone finally picked it up. "Operator Number Two," an overly cheerful voice said.

"Hello, Number Two," I mumbled back into the phone's mouthpiece. "This is Dr. Marion. Somebody paged me."

"Dr. Marion?" the operator asked. "Did anyone page Dr. Marion?" I could hear confused voices on the other end of the phone, and the conversation seemed to go on forever. I began banging my fist weakly against the telephone table as I impatiently waited for something to happen. Finally, Operator Number Two came back on: "Dr. Marion, call eight-zero-eight-five."

I pushed down the button on the receiver cradle and quickly dialed the number of the general pediatric ward. "Please let this be something I can handle over the phone," I prayed as I waited for someone to answer. Ginny, the ward clerk, picked up the phone on the fourth ring: "General pediatrics," she said in her usual cheerful voice.

"Hi," I said. "This is Bob. Somebody wants me?"

"Yes, Dr. Marion," the ward clerk replied. "Dr. Donahue is here. He wants to see you right away."

I sighed. "I'm kind of busy right now," I lied to the clerk. "Could you ask if he'd speak to me over the phone?"

There were a few moments when I heard muffled voices in the background, and then Ginny came back on: "No, he wants you to come to the ward right now. Those are his specific orders."

"For Christ's sake!" I shouted. I sighed, pausing a few seconds before I realized there was no way out. "Okay, I'll be there in a couple of minutes," I said at last, just before slamming the receiver down.

Cursing, I retrieved my socks and pulled them back on over my unwashed feet. "Cardiologists you can talk to over the phone," I muttered as I reknotted my tie over the blue shirt I'd been wearing nonstop since early the previous morning, a shirt that had been stained by my sweat and the blood shed by my patients during the long night. "Endocrinologists you can talk to over the phone," I added as I gazed at my sickly, pale green reflection in the tiny mirror mounted over the phone table and tried, using my fingers, to reassemble my hair into an orderly pattern. "Even neurologists you can talk to over the phone. But for oncologists, you have to be there; they have to see you in person or they don't believe they're really speaking to you." I laced up my sneakers. "They're nauseating, every one of them." Angrily, I kicked open the door of the on-call room and, squinting to adjust to the light in the hall, began to make my way back to the general pediatric ward. "I hate them all!"

I saw him as soon as I reached the door to the ward. He was standing near the nurses' station; in fact, it seemed everyone was standing down there, forming a crowd huddled around the director of pediatric hematology and oncology, a mass of humanity composed of Cindy and Andrea, my fellow interns, Ted, the senior resident, as well as the fellows, residents, medical students, and nurse practitioners who formed the hematology/oncology team. It looked as though the ward's complete day shift of staff nurses had also been assembled, and even some parents of patients, many of whom I barely recognized from the night before, whose names I couldn't quite recall, were standing around Dr. Donahue as if they'd been posed. Having no idea what was going on, not comprehending what was about to happen, I approached this tableau, like a lamb going to slaughter, without a bit of reluctance or a moment's hesitation.

Dr. Kevin Donahue, professor of pediatrics and the director of pediatric hematology and oncology at the Boston Medical Center, had been, back in the early sixties, an internationally known presence in academic medicine. He had made his reputation with the pioneering research he'd done on the care and management of children with acute lymphoblastic leukemia, or ALL as it is usually called. Back at the start of Dr. Donahue's career, ALL had been a uniformly lethal disease, a dreaded killer of over four thousand children in the United States every year. Dr. Donahue and his fellow oncologists had waged war on ALL, gradually developing an armamentarium of chemotherapeutic agents and working out protocols on how, when, in what doses, and on whom these drugs should be used. And they had won: for the first time, using these new chemicals, physicians could treat their young patients with leukemia and control the course of the disease. Suddenly, thanks to the work of Dr. Donahue and his colleagues, the majority of children afflicted with ALL were no longer dying of the effects of their disease but were able to survive into adulthood.

In the early sixties Kevin Donahue had been one of the brightest stars in pediatrics, but over the ensuing years his star had dimmed dramatically. Since the completion of his successful research, Dr. Donahue had become stalled, unable to repeat the quality of work he'd performed at the start of his career, incapable of living up to the expectations the medical community had of him. By the time I began my internship he was in his mid-fifties but looked much older—because, the grapevine had it, of a combination of factors; including his ineffectiveness as a researcher, his three failed marriages, the aggravation and grief caused by being a physician who had spent his career dealing with hundreds of critically ill children and adolescents and their families, and most significant, his years of alcoholism. I was thinking of none of this as I approached the nurses' station that morning in January; I was too angry and too tired to dwell on anything other than the fact that once again I'd been abused by one of the people in charge.

Dr. Donahue, who had white hair and a heavily lined face, was tall and thin and stood straight as a stick. As usual, he was dressed in a long, heavily starched, spot-lessly clean white coat. The overall effect of his bearing and clothing was that he resembled the prototypical senior doctor on a television soap opera. As I came closer, I saw that he appeared to be furious. I made it to within five feet of him before he started to let me have it: "Dr. Marion, how nice of you to show up! I understand you were off taking a nap. I hope my needing to speak with you hasn't inconvenienced you all that much."

I didn't answer. My tired brain, which had long before begun to fail in its ability to synthesize creative thought, was not processing this incoming information rapidly enough; not being able to come up with a snappy reply, I remained silent. Obviously a little disappointed by my unresponsiveness, the oncologist continued: "I believe you admitted one of our patients yesterday afternoon, a young man named Richard Cannon. Do you happen to recall admitting Mr. Cannon?"

I nodded, my memory slowly fixing back on the previous afternoon. "Sure, the twenty-year-old with osteogenic sarcoma," I replied, naming a malignant cancer of the bone. The young man, a junior at Boston University, had first presented intense pain in his right leg at the age of fourteen; back then, after the cancer had been diagnosed, his leg was amputated above the knee, he had undergone an intensive course of radiation therapy, and the oncologists believed they'd effected a cure. But during the previous summer Richard had developed a cough that simply wouldn't go away; a chest X ray revealed lesions in both lungs, apparently metastases from his long-indolent cancer. He returned to Dr. Donahue's clinic and was immediately put on chemotherapy.

"Well, good," Dr. Donahue continued condescendingly. "It's good to see that at least you have the ability to remember something about yesterday. Dr. Marion, do you recall why Mr. Cannon was admitted?"

"I was told that he was having some respiratory distress," I replied. "He was fine by the time he reached the floor, though. I wasn't sure exactly why he needed to be here."

"You don't have any idea why we were concerned about him?" Dr. Donahue asked.

I paused. "Well, maybe you were concerned that he might have come down with a slight case of pneumonia."

"No, we weren't concerned about pneumonia," the attending physician said, shaking his head from side to side. "He had no fever. Didn't one of our fellows ask you to order a special test for this patient?"

I thought for a moment. "Yeah," I finally answered. "I was told to get an echocardiogram done."

"That's right," Donahue said. "Now, why in the world do you think we might have wanted to get an echocardiogram on Mr. Cannon?"

I thought again, coming up completely blank. When enough time had passed and I had made no attempt to answer, Dr. Donahue gave me what he must have thought was an excellent hint: "He's being treated with daunomycin, Dr. Marion."

My exhausted memory banks drew another blank. "I guess you must have been worried about some kind of heart damage," I attempted, knowing at least that echocardiograms provided an ultrasonic view of the functioning of the heart.

"Very good, Dr. Marion," Donahue replied. "Whenever one of our patients on daunomycin has any kind of respiratory difficulty, we're always concerned about the presence of a pericardial effusion, which is a side effect of the drug. We always admit these patients to the hospital for careful observation, and perform echocardiograms on them. If we document the presence of a fluid collection in the pericardium surrounding the heart, it must be drained at once, or else the patient's cardiac function might be compromised and the patient could die. Tell me, Dr. Marion: did Richard Cannon's echocardiogram show that he had a pericardial fluid collection?"

When I saw at last where all this was leading, I felt like crying. "I don't know," I said. "I never got a chance to check the results of the echocardiogram."

A smile came to the oncologist's wrinkled face. "You didn't check the echocardiogram? You have a patient who might have a pericardial effusion, whose life might be hanging in the balance, and you didn't even check the results of this one measly test?"

He stopped, I guess to give me a chance to come up with some excuse or other, but I remained silent. He had me, I had to admit. I had screwed up, and nothing I could say would make things right. Dr. Donahue continued: "This patient could have died, do you know that? If Mr. Cannon had had a pericardial effusion and died, it would have been your fault, because you had better things to do than make a simple phone call to the radiologist." He hesitated a moment and then, shaking his head, concluded: "Dr. Marion, how can you even call yourself a doctor?"

I stood there, still silent. All the fight had been beaten out of me; all those nights on call spent without any sleep, all those admissions to the ICU, all those children who had died had taken their toll. I stiffened my lip and fought back the tears that were trying to form in my eyes. I didn't want to cry, not in front of the whole ward team and the oncologists, and all those nurses and parents. I didn't want to give Dr. Donahue that satisfaction, the pleasure of chalking up yet another intern whom he'd been able to bring to tears through his bullying. So I stood there, rigid, while he shook his white head in silence. He then turned and walked down the hall, the parade of oncologists following along behind him. When they were finally gone, before Andrea or Cindy or Ted, who had stood by watching, stunned, while this terrible exchange occurred, unable themselves to believe it was happening and equally unable to do anything to stop it, could reach me, I bolted; I ran down the hall, off the ward, to the on-call room. Once inside I closed the door and, lying back on the upper bunk in the silent darkness, did some serious thinking.

Something was wrong with this place; some serious deficiency had to be present in any training program that would allow an attending physician to destroy an intern in public the way Kevin Donahue had just destroyed me. There was no question that I'd made a mistake—although Richard Cannon had seemed healthy and was breathing comfortably from the moment I admitted him to the general pediatric ward, I had been given a plan to follow and I hadn't followed it. I had been wrong and I deserved to be disciplined. But I didn't deserve to be humiliated.

Never in my four years of medical school had I witnessed a scene like the one that had just occurred on the general pediatric ward; I'd never seen or heard of a single intern at Jonas Bronck Hospital who'd been yelled at in front of a crowd of people by an attending physician. Now, having just recently made it to the halfway point in my internship, I had not only witnessed such scenes numerous times, as other attendings found fault with and attacked my fellow interns; now I myself had become one of the victims. Lying on that bunk bed, the thought occurred to me for the first time that maybe the fault didn't lie with me; maybe all the bad feelings I'd been experiencing during the previous six months, the anger and hostility, the depression and lethargy, the realization that something had been missing in my life, hadn't been due to my personal failings or incompetence, as I'd come to believe; maybe they stemmed from the attitudes that permeated this hospital. With that realization in the on-call room that morning in January, I made my decision: come next July, regardless of what I had to do or where I would have to go, I would not return to the Boston Medical Center to work as a junior resident.

That afternoon I called Alan Cozza, the director of pediatrics at Jonas Bronck Hospital, a man I'd come to know during my fourth year of medical school, and told him everything that had happened to me over the past few months. Alan promptly offered me a job as a junior resident at Jonas Bronck beginning the next July. I accepted without hesitation; come summer, Beth and I would be returning to New York. Now I only had to survive the last half of internship, and our marriage had to survive the next six months. Neither goal was going to be easy to accomplish.

11

Beth's Heart Attack

**Eighth month of internship,
February 1979**

"Bob, wake up."

I heard the words, and felt the elbow jabbing sharply into my ribs, but I decided to ignore them. I didn't want to be interrupted just then, not at that wonderful moment. I'd been standing somewhere within the lush confines of the Boston Public Garden. It was a beautiful summer morning: the temperature was in the high seventies and there was a soft, warm breeze coming off the pond and blowing gently against my face; I felt more relaxed and happier than I had in months. Off in the distance, on one of the swan boats, I could clearly make out a tall, thin man with white hair and a heavily lined face who was standing up in the boat, waving his arms wildly in the air. It didn't take me long to recognize this figure, who was wearing a heavily starched, luminously white, knee-length doctor's coat and a sour expression on his face, as the director of pediatric hematology and oncology at the Boston Medical Center, Dr. Kevin Donahue. Looking down at my right hand, I saw that I just happened to be carrying a semiautomatic assault weapon—not the sort of equipment I usually brought along on leisurely trips to the park. Lifting the gun's sighting mechanism to my right eye and honing in on the target, I was just beginning to squeeze the trigger with my index finger when I was once more disturbed by one of those irritating jabs to my ribs. Again I heard these words: "Bob, wake up!"

Opening my eyes just enough to catch a glimpse of Beth, who was wide awake and sitting up against the headboard on her side of the bed, I made a low-pitched moaning noise, a feeble attempt at saying the word "What?"

"Bob, wake up," she said again, her voice panicked. "I think I'm having a heart attack."

I roused myself enough to respond in a language understandable to other human beings. "A heart attack! There's no way you could be having a heart attack. You're only twenty-six years old; that's much too young to be having heart disease. It's probably just gas or something. Try to go back to sleep!"

A few seconds passed, and suddenly there I was, back in the Public Garden; I had returned to the exact moment when I had Donahue's craggy, mean face clearly within my sights; I was again getting ready to squeeze the trigger of the rifle when that elbow stuck itself into my ribs again. "Bob, this isn't like any pain I've ever had before," Beth said when I reluctantly raised my head from the pillow. "I really think I'm having a heart attack. It hurts really bad. You have to get up and take me to the emergency room."

"The emergency room!" I shouted, rolling over onto my back and sitting up. "What the hell are you talking about? Where does it hurt?" I switched on the lamp on the night table. "Show me exactly where the pain is."

"Over here," Beth answered, outlining with her right hand the entire left side of her chest.

"Is it a dull pain or a sharp pain?" I asked automatically, shifting easily from sleeping husband to overtired intern, and relying on the questions I had been taught to ask patients when they presented with complaints such as this.

"Sharp," she said. "Like someone is sticking a knife into my breast."

"Are you having any shortness of breath?"

"A little," she responded meekly. "It hurts when I breathe in deeply. That's what's really got me worried."

"Does the pain stay in one place, or does it radiate?" I continued objectively, not revealing any emotion about the fact that my wife was obviously frightened to death.

"It kind of goes up into my arm," she replied, now rubbing her left shoulder with the fingers of her right hand.

"Well, it's probably nothing more than musculoskeletal pain," I said, trying to stifle a yawn. "The best thing to do for musculoskeletal pain is to get a lot of rest. My advice is to take some aspirin and try to go back to sleep. I'm sure you'll feel better in the morning. If it's not better by tomorrow, you should go to see a doctor." With that, I turned off the light and rolled back onto my left side.

Pretty soon I was at something that looked like a county fair. I was standing at one of those booths where you try to knock a clown into a pool of water, only instead of a clown, Dr. Donahue, still wearing that long white coat and that angry expression, was seated up on the chair. Eager to have a turn, I hastily handed the person in charge, who bore a striking resemblance to Ginny, the clerk on the general pediatric ward, a handful of change. Rather than handing me three baseballs in return, the ward clerk gave me three beepers of the type used at the Boston Medical Center. I was just getting ready to launch the first beeper in the direction of the chief of hematology and oncology when I felt that elbow digging into my ribs yet again and heard those now familiar words: "Bob, wake up."

"What now?" I asked, trying my best to sound sympathetic but failing miserably.

"I took two aspirin and I tried to go back to sleep," Beth said, now almost in tears, "but the pain's not getting any better. In fact, it's getting worse. I really think I'm having a heart attack.''

I sighed. ''You realize I was on call last night, don't you?'' I shot back at her. ''You realize I was working in the emergency room alone, without any backup, and that I didn't get a wink of sleep. You realize this is my only chance to get some rest, don't you?'' Her response, a nod of her head and tears filling her eyes, was too much for me to bear. Even though she didn't say a word, I knew there was no way out. So, reluctantly, I hoisted myself out of bed.

So far it hadn't exactly been what you'd call a terrific year for either Beth or our marriage. At the start of my internship, while I'd been getting my mail (mostly circulars from local supermarkets and bills) and spending spare moments now and then at the apartment in Watertown, Beth was living in New York in a tiny dormitory room on the Columbia campus. Still involved in the laboratory experiments that, she hoped, would eventually form the foundation of her dissertation in molecular biology, her work had become stalled, mired in the misery that our existence had become.

The commuting between Boston and New York had proved to be a major problem. During July, August, and September our lives went something like this: we'd both work all week in our separate cities, then on Friday afternoon or Saturday morning, Beth would take a shuttle flight up to Boston. I rarely volunteered to make the trip down to New York during this period; having come off a thirty-six-hour shift or getting ready to start one, I always claimed to be too tired or too damned depressed to travel.

But then, sometime toward the middle of October, Beth started having severe, burning pains in the center of her abdomen. The pains came and went at odd hours of the day or night, but they occurred frequently enough for her to become concerned. When she became convinced that something was definitely wrong, she made an appointment with the student health service physician at Columbia. After hearing her story, that doctor ordered an upper gastrointestinal series. The test was enough to diagnose the problem: Beth had developed a peptic ulcer.

Now although I'm the first to admit that I've got my faults, most of our friends would tell you that I'm a reasonably good husband. If Beth had gotten her ulcer under normal circumstances I would have been sympathetic and understanding; I would have tried to take time off from work in order to help nurse her back to health; I would have made sure that she ate the right foods and took Tagamet, a drug decreasing the amount of hydrochloric acid produced by the stomach, which the health service doctor had prescribed for her. But Beth didn't get her ulcer under normal circumstances; she got it right in the middle of my internship. By that October I was already so exhausted and emotionally wrecked that I couldn't possibly have been sympathetic or understanding about my wife's—or for that matter anyone else's—ailments. Instead, I actually responded with rage at the malicious act that had been perpetrated against me: "What the hell right does she have getting an ulcer?" I asked myself after Beth told me the results of her upper GI series. "I'm the one who's under all the fucking stress! I deserve that ulcer, not her! How dare she take it away from me?"

But of course Beth too had been under a great deal of stress. I didn't learn this until much later, but my wife has a tremendous, irrational fear of flying. Taking the shuttle back and forth between New York and Boston every weekend had wreaked havoc on her gastrointestinal tract, not to speak of how it interfered with every phase of her life, including her work in the lab. One Sunday afternoon in November, therefore, after another weekend spent discussing our very limited options, Beth decided to take a leave of absence from graduate school for the remainder of the academic year. Since that time we had been living together in Boston. Between the medication and the elimination of the underlying cause of her stress, Beth's symptoms had come under control, and she was happy again. For my part, however, I was just as crazed and unbalanced as I'd been since July. It now was February, and in the middle of the night Beth had come up with a brand-new complaint; she was sure she was having a heart attack. Exhausted, numb, and half-asleep, I had no option other than getting up and taking her to the emergency room at the Boston Medical Center.

I got out of bed and began to get dressed, mumbling, "She thinks *she's* having a heart attack!" under my breath the whole while. I bundled into my parka, and as we walked out into the sub-zero-degree early morning air and started to make our way across the parking lot to our car, I sighed, just loud enough for Beth to hear, "Oh, well. No sleep last night, no sleep tonight, probably no sleep tomorrow night." All during the seven-mile trip to the hospital I kept up a constant, barely audible monologue about some of the terrible, violent things that interns and residents were reported to have done when they hadn't been allowed to get an adequate amount of rest. All the while Beth sat quietly, clutching at her chest, trying hard to catch her breath.

We were about a block away from the hospital parking lot when Beth decided to add what might be considered an important piece of historical information. "Do you think this pain might have anything to do with the fact that I jogged five miles this morning?" she asked.

"You jogged five miles this morning?" I said, so startled by this revelation that I momentarily took my eyes off the road and almost drove the car into a snowbank.

"Yeah," she replied a little hesitantly. "I've been thinking I need to get more exercise, so I decided to take up jogging. I ran from our apartment building to Watertown Square and back again. I just thought about it. Do you think the running might have anything to do with this pain?"

I tried to control myself, to hold back—I really did. But I couldn't help it; I was just too weak. "You decide that all of the sudden, out of the clear blue, it might be a good idea to take up jogging, and on the very first day, you run five miles. And then, that same night, you begin to feel sharp, shooting pains in the left side of your chest. You wake me up out of a sound sleep and force me to take you to the goddamn emergency room because you think you're having a heart attack, and now you want to know if I think that maybe your jogging had anything to do with the pain in your chest? No, what a silly thing to think, of course your jogging has nothing to do with your chest pain! In the entire history of the world, no one, not a single person, has ever been known to have any pain in their chest or their arms or their legs after the first time they've gone jogging. It's all obviously just a ridiculous coincidence!''

By then I was pulling the car into the parking lot. Beth sheepishly said, ''Bob, maybe we ought to just go home.''

''No way!'' I was almost yelling. ''I'm not leaving now. I want you to tell this story to the guy who's on call in the emergency room tonight. I want to hear what he has to say about it. I've come this far; I deserve at least one good laugh!''

We walked through the emergency room entrance in silence punctuated only by my whispering *''Jogging!''* under my breath, followed by a snicker or two. The ER was deathly quiet, and the nurse who met us at the triage desk took Beth in at once. Because of her complaint, the nurse did a stat electrocardiogram. Afterward, Beth was placed in one of the treatment rooms, where we sat, waiting for the physician on call that night to arrive.

The doctor, a woman named Ellen Smith, came in about ten minutes later. Paying no attention whatever to Beth, she initially seemed completely absorbed in the long, thin strip of paper on which the electrocardiogram had been recorded. After a minute or two of complete silence, Ellen, whom I knew from my nights on call in this same emergency room, nodded toward me and introduced herself to Beth. She started taking a history, asking virtually the same questions I had asked when Beth first wrenched me away from that wonderful dream. This time, without prompting, Beth volunteered the information about her five-mile run that morning, figuring, I guess, that if she told all the facts Ellen might not give her too hard a time. But this bit of data which I had thought so important didn't elicit any response from the emergency room resident: she remained serious, a concerned expression on her face.

After completing her questions, Ellen took the stethoscope that was dangling around her neck and carefully examined Beth's chest. She listened at every possible position for a good ten minutes before putting the instrument down again. Then she asked a few more questions: "Have you ever blacked out?"

"No," Beth replied.

"Do you ever get a fluttering feeling in your chest?"

"Yes," Beth answered. "All the time."

"Do you notice when it happens most?"

Beth thought for a few moments. "Usually in the morning, I guess."

"After you've drunk coffee?" the resident asked.

"Yes. Now that you mention it, it always happens right after I've had a cup or two of coffee."

"Wait a minute," I broke in, now getting concerned myself. "Why are you asking all these questions? Is there something wrong?"

"Well, I'm not exactly sure. Look at this rhythm strip." She handed me part of the long strip of paper on which the electrocardiogram was recorded. As I scanned the squiggly lines that covered the thing from one end to the other, the resident continued: "As you can see, there are lots of premature contractions, at least ten a minute. Some part of her heart is beating earlier than it should, as if it wasn't part of the regular conducting system. You see that, don't you?"

I nodded but didn't utter a sound. Ellen now spoke directly to Beth: "The premature contractions appear to be atrial in origin, so I'm not too concerned about them. But your pulse is very irregular and I think I hear an unusual heart sound, called an S-two click. These findings are frequently seen in a condition called mitral valve prolapse. I don't think it's anything serious, but it definitely needs to be investigated further.''

"You mean she's really got pathology?'' I asked.

"I can't be sure,'' the ER doctor said in my direction. "I'm just saying it needs to be checked out further.'' She continued to Beth: "You should call a cardiologist in the morning and arrange for an echocardiogram to be done as soon as possible. Do you have any questions?''

Neither of us did, and after saying, "Well, nice meeting you,'' Ellen Smith departed, leaving us alone in silence.

I remained silent all the way home. I could just barely hear Beth, sitting in the passenger seat, muttering softly under her breath somewhere to the right of me: "He was on call last night, and he hasn't gotten enough sleep; he's always complaining about one thing or another. But I'm the one with real pathology. A heart condition, that's what I've got, but he's too damned busy to get out of bed and take me to the hospital.''

We made it home at a little after four in the morning. I did manage to get an hour and a half of sleep, but it wasn't nearly enough; completely exhausted, I limped through the next day, doing my work at no more than half power.

That morning Beth called one of the cardiologists who had been recommended by the triage nurse in the emergency room, making an appointment for a complete examination a few days later. The cardiologist confirmed Ellen Smith's findings, hearing an S-2 click and seeing the premature contractions on another electrocardiogram strip. An echocardiogram was then done, an ultrasound examination of the workings of Beth's heart, which revealed that she did in fact have a mild case of mitral valve prolapse, an abnormality in the valve that separates the left atrium from the left ventricle. The condition wouldn't affect her overall health. She would need to take antibiotics whenever she had dental work done, but that would be the extent of the effect of her mitral valve prolapse on her life.

It didn't matter that the pain Beth had experienced that night hadn't in any way been caused by her "heart condition," as she now refers to it. The pain clearly resulted from a muscle sprain in her rib cage, an injury related to her jogging which gradually resolved over the days following our middle-of-the-night visit to the emergency room. It didn't matter that I had been correct in my diagnosis of musculoskeletal pain, and that, at least technically, she'd been wrong. What was ultimately important was that the symptoms of chest pain of which Beth complained had led directly to a diagnostic workup and the discovery of a minor abnormality in her heart. What really mattered, the final take-home lesson of this story, was that, in private life as well as professional, I was an intern and interns are always wrong!

How far I'd come; how low I'd fallen. From the student who had fought to get into medical school because, naively, he wanted to do something with his life that might help his fellow man, I had, in just four and a half years, been transformed into a creature unable to care for, or to feel sympathy or empathy for, any other human being. Between January and about May of 1979, the exhaustion and stress that circumscribed my life on all sides during my internship had changed me into a frightening, unfeeling monster. It was a transformation that both Beth and I were afraid might be permanent.

As best as I can recall, I moved through those first few months of 1979 in a state resembling suspended animation. I was an automaton, having no feelings, not giving any thought to what I was doing or why. I woke up every morning, went to work, did what I had to do, and came home, only to go back to sleep immediately. Beth and I had no social life during that period; we never went out, never visited with friends or neighbors, never did anything enjoyable. To me, life was nothing more than too much work intermingled with not nearly enough sleep.

My automaton personality of those difficult months colored my reactions in the middle of March, when Beth and I attended a wedding in New York. Things happened during that wedding which changed people's lives, but none of the events of the day had any effect on me.

12

A Wedding

**Ninth month of internship,
March 1979**

I stared at the fruit cup for what must have been an hour.
I didn't eat it; I just sat, staring down into the crystal
bowl, wishing that, instead of the first course of dinner,
it was a nice, soft, warm bed. I wasn't at all hungry that
afternoon, but I sure was tired; all I wanted to do was
go to sleep, but I knew I wasn't going to be able to do
that for a long time. Beth and I were back in New York,
at least temporarily, at a place called Terrace on the Park,
attending the wedding reception of two people I'd never
in my life seen before.

It was the second Sunday in March; I had been on call
the day before and was up the entire previous night,
working on the infectious disease ward. During the past
few weeks a large number of children in the Boston area
had come down with viral meningitis, and the entire ward
was filled with irritable, febrile kids with stiff necks who
all required close and careful observation. The work kept
me on my feet, running for twenty-four hours straight,
and when Ray Eastman, the intern who had come to relieve me, arrived at a little after eight o'clock that Sunday
morning, I wasn't fit to do anything other than go home
and get into bed. But that didn't matter: Beth and I had
accepted the invitation to attend this wedding. So, after

signing the ward out to Ray, I took a car from the medical center directly to Logan Airport, where I met Beth, and together we caught the ten o'clock Eastern shuttle bound for La Guardia.

It wasn't a terrific flight; the plane bumped and jerked all the way from Boston to New York, and I developed a case of motion sickness. I had hoped to get some sleep during the flight, but the plane's unsteadiness made that impossible. By the time we met Beth's father, who had come to pick us up, outside the shuttle terminal building, going to this or any wedding was about the last thing in the world I wanted to do. My father-in-law drove us directly to the catering hall, a huge structure located just across the highway from the airport, and while Beth changed her clothes in the bride's room, I went into one of the men's rooms, washed and shaved my face, and changed from my smelly on-call clothes into the suit Beth had packed for me before she left our apartment that morning. After a few minutes of composing myself, now fully dressed but still feeling horrible, I joined Beth and her family in the chapel and waited for the ceremony to begin.

The bride was Beth's second cousin. They hadn't seen each other in more than ten years; as far as I was concerned, they'd picked a pretty lousy time to have a reunion. But Beth had been eager to come, so, without too much complaining, I settled myself down on one of the chapel's hard-backed pews and tried desperately to stay awake while the rabbi rambled on about the two strangers standing at the front of the room. I don't think I did too badly during the ceremony, considering my exhausted state: I only fell asleep twice. Beth told me afterward that she wouldn't have awakened me either, except that my snoring had begun to drown out the rabbi's voice.

After the ceremony ended the entire party was led into the dining room. Beth directed me to our assigned table, one located near the bandstand, and she sat me on a chair, between her and her mother. And I stared down at my fruit cup, completely undisturbed, for a hell of a long time. Thankfully, no one came over to meet me, no one talked to me, no one bothered me at all until a waitress appeared, tapped me on the shoulder, and asked if I was finished with the fruit. When I didn't answer, the crystal bowl that had been monopolizing my attention for such a long time at last disappeared. All things considered, I figured I was doing all right; *I can survive this*, I thought to myself, *as long as no one expects too much from me*.

But then the band started playing a horah. The music was so loud that I could feel the fillings vibrate in my teeth. On hearing the melody, many of the guests rose from their chairs, formed a circle in the center of the floor, and began the traditional dance. The bandleader, however, was apparently not satisfied with the crowd's response. "I still see some people in their seats!" he shouted into the microphone. "I want to see everybody up and dancing!"

His request brought a few more people to their feet, but I wasn't about to budge. "I said everybody!" the guy repeated, this time pointing his finger directly at our table. Beth, a little embarrassed by the bandleader's attention, started to rise and pulled me by the hand. Without putting up much of a fight, I allowed her to lead me into the circle.

I saw the man go down. He was old and obese, and he shouldn't have been dancing as vigorously as he had been. I was on him almost before he hit the ground. It was all reflex; I was so numb that it couldn't have been anything else.

Feeling around on the right side of the man's neck, I attempted to palpate the pulse in his carotid artery, but no pulse was present. My father-in-law, a doctor himself, reached the man nearly as quickly as I had, and as I went for the chest, he cleared the man's airway. Automatically I began external cardiac compressions, pushing down firmly on the upper part of the man's breastbone with the heels of my hands and repeatedly counting *one, one thousand, two, one thousand, three, one thousand, four, one thousand, five, one thousand,* out loud, as I had been trained to do in the basic cardiac life support course I'd taken at the start of my internship. In synch with my actions, my father-in-law began administering mouth-to-mouth resuscitation, blowing air into the man's mouth every time I reached *five, one thousand.*

Off to the side of my consciousness, I was aware that the band had stopped playing and that a crowd had formed around us, the guests at first curious about what was happening, then filled with morbid fascination as the drama continued to unfold. At one point, someone said he had called the local rescue squad; at another, Beth helped me slip off my suit jacket, and I was pumping in my shirtsleeves. But these events were incidental: I was concentrating everything I had left on that man's condition. He looked okay, his skin pink and lifelike, as long as I pushed down hard on his sternum and my father-in-law breathed air into his lungs. But whenever I stopped to feel for a pulse, or my father-in-law stopped to catch his breath, there was nothing. For all intents and purposes, the man was dead the moment he hit the ground.

Thinking back on it, I have realized that the outcome might have been different if the hall had been equipped with resuscitation equipment. The man might have survived if we had been able to start an intravenous line and shoot some medications into him. But at the time, nothing like that was available: no drugs, no intravenous solution, no ambu bags, no needles. So it came down to my father-in-law and me, breathing and pumping, breathing and pumping, over and over again, until the members of the rescue squad finally arrived. Sadly, we just weren't enough.

There were two guys, and they carried their equipment in fishing tackle boxes. On arriving, they immediately slid a wooden board under the man's back to facilitate the cardiopulmonary resuscitation then under way, and the paramedic who seemed to be in charge felt for a pulse. "How long has this been going on?" he asked.

"I don't know," I replied, standing by while the paramedic checked for a pulse. "Seems like forever."

One of the other guests said that it had been a total of fifteen minutes since the music stopped.

"Do you want to try to shock him?" the head paramedic asked. His assistant shrugged his shoulders, and as I continued to compress the man's sternum and my father-in-law to deliver mouth-to-mouth resuscitation, the paramedics broke out their portable cardioverter, a device that, when triggered, delivers an electric shock to the chest. The assistant paramedic turned on the machine and placed its plastic paddles against the man's chest. I stopped my work. The paramedics, my father-in-law, and I all looked toward the cardiac monitor screen that was mounted on the face of the cardioverter; none of us were surprised to see it register a flatline.

"Is it charged?" the first paramedic asked. The other one nodded. "Okay, let 'er rip!"

"Everybody off!" the second paramedic ordered. When he was sure neither my father-in-law nor I was in contact with the body, he pushed a button on the face of the cardioverter: the dead man's back arched a few inches up off the floor as the machine discharged its voltage, but when the head paramedic checked for a pulse, he shook his head and said, "We better try 'er again."

The second paramedic recharged the paddles and shouted once more, "Everybody off!" His command wasn't necessary this time: no one was even close to the body. The second paramedic again pushed the button on the paddle, and again the man's back arched up off the dance floor; but again, when the head paramedic palpated the man's neck, no blood could be felt coursing through the carotid artery. "What do you say we get him the hell out of here now?" the head paramedic asked quietly. His assistant silently nodded.

As they lifted the dead man off the wooden board and onto a stretcher, the paramedics told my father-in-law and me to continue our resuscitation efforts. We moved as one, the four of us rolling the stretcher out of the room and through the lobby, out through the elegant entrance to the hall, and onto the sidewalk. The ambulance was parked at the curb. When we reached the door of the wagon, the head paramedic said we could stop. "You know he's dead," he added.

"I know," I replied. "He was gone the second he hit the ground."

"I didn't think it would be such a good idea to declare him in the middle of all that," the guy went on, pointing back to the reception hall. "What's going on in there, a wedding?"

I nodded.

"This guy a relative?"

"Yeah," my father-in-law answered. "He's the groom's uncle."

"It's not such a good sign," the assistant paramedic observed, "having your uncle die on the day you get married."

They finished putting the body into the back of the ambulance and climbed in to drive away. After watching the wagon drive off, its sirens screaming, my father-in-law and I went to the men's room, the one in which I'd changed into my suit a few hours before, and attempted to clean ourselves up. "Are you okay?" my father-in-law asked.

"Yeah, I'm fine," I replied. "Just a little tired, I guess."

In a few minutes we headed back into the reception hall, where, to my astonishment, the party had resumed at full tilt. Dinner was being served, but I still didn't feel hungry; I just stared down at the plate of roast beef and little potatoes which had been placed in front of me for what seemed like another hour. After a long time had passed, I turned to Beth and asked if she didn't think it was starting to get very late. She said she thought it would be all right for us to leave, and after saying goodbye to the bride and groom (I had to reintroduce myself to them, so that they knew who I was), Beth's father drove us back to the airport. We caught the shuttle back to Boston, and after landing at Logan, Beth drove back to our apartment in Watertown. I was in bed by nine-thirty that night, and I slept soundly until six the next morning, when I had to return to the infectious disease ward to continue the battle against the epidemic of viral meningitis.

I went through much of the second half of my internship as if I was under the influence of a long-acting general anesthetic. I have almost no memories of those months; although some terrible events occurred in the lives of my patients during that time, I've managed to repress almost everything. The second half of my internship damaged me, destroying the last vestiges of humanism that survived from my medical school days.

But then, sometime in May, the anesthetic began to wear off. As the end of my internship year drew closer, I slowly began to wake up. One of the first things I remember from that period was the death of one of my patients, Tom Costello.

13

When Tom Died

**Eleventh month of internship,
May 1979**

The Tom Costello who died in May wasn't anything like the
Tom Costello I had come to know back in September,
during my first rotation on the general pediatric ward at
the Boston Medical Center. That Tom, who had been
admitted near the end of my third month of internship,
was a husky, active twelve-year-old who seemed far too
healthy to be an inpatient in any hospital. When he first
came onto the ward, I remember thinking that some mistake had been made, that the wrong child had been sent
to the medical center for admission; but then, as I sat at
his bedside and listened to the history of the present illness that he reluctantly recounted for me, I began to understand the reason for the look of deep concern on his
mother's face.

He'd been losing some weight, the boy told me, and
had been feeling kind of run down. Although he'd spent
the beginning of the summer heavily involved in his favorite pastime, playing second base on one of the local
Little League teams, Tom began missing games during
August: he said he had simply been too tired to play,
having the stamina to field his position for only two or
three innings at a time. Then, as September rolled
around, he began experiencing vague aches and pains in

156

the joints of his legs and shoulders. But he and his mother tried to deny that anything was seriously wrong; Mrs. Costello believed that her son's uncharacteristic lethargy was nothing more than a reaction to the unusually long heat wave that had gripped the Boston area during August; she also assumed that the joint pains Tom had been having were due to the rapid drop in temperature which occurred as summer drew to a close. But then, on the morning prior to his admission to the hospital, while Tom was brushing his teeth, his gums began to bleed; the hemorrhaging, which the Costellos described as heavy, continued for well over an hour. It was followed by periodic oozing from Tom's mouth through most of the rest of that day; the trickle of blood simply didn't want to stop. The boy's mother, suddenly growing very concerned, immediately called Tom's pediatrician. The doctor wasted no time in admitting the boy to the hospital. Tom's acute lymphoblastic leukemia was diagnosed his first day on the ward.

During the remainder of that month's rotation on the general pediatric ward I spent a lot of hours in Tom's room. I felt sorry for the boy; he seemed like a nice kid, and his prognosis had been horrible. I also found that Tom and I shared a major interest: we were both ardent baseball fans. On the very first day he was in the hospital, I noticed a Boston Red Sox cap on the boy's bedside table. "Do you like the Sox?" I asked, just trying to make conversation.

"Doesn't everybody?" he answered.

I smiled and said, "Well, you know, I'm originally from the Bronx . . ."

"You're not a Yankees fan, are you?" Tom asked in disgust, and I nodded.

That September, all of Boston was gripped by pennant fever. The Yankees and the Red Sox, a notoriously fanatic baseball rivalry, were neck and neck in the standings in the American League's eastern division. When Tom was admitted to the hospital the Yankees held a slight edge, but they seemed to be fading fast, raising the spirits of Tom and all the other Red Sox crazies who inhabited the city. I had been keeping my long-standing allegiance to the Yankees a secret since being a New York fan in Boston at a time like that could prove somewhat dangerous, but I figured I would level with Tom; I wanted to see how he'd take it.

He reacted the way most normal twelve-year-olds would: he shook his head slowly, rolled his eyes, and smiled slightly. "My doctor's a Yankees fan!" he said sadly. "How embarrassing!"

We spent a great deal of time after that talking about the rival teams. I saw a lot of myself in Tom. He let me know very quickly that his favorite player was Carl Yastrzemski, whom he idolized. He had memorized every possible statistic about Yaz, from his lifetime batting average to his birthday, his fielding percentage to his parents' and grandparents' names and occupations. I smiled as I listened to him spout off facts and statistics about his hero: it reminded me of my own preadolescent obsession with Mickey Mantle, for whom, between the ages of seven and thirteen, I'd lived and breathed.

Despite my obviously severe psychiatric disturbance— the only possible explanation, Tom must have figured, for my undying loyalty to the odious Yankees—I was accepted as a true and deserving baseball fan; during the last day I worked on the ward, he invited me to watch the Red Sox game on television with him. Though I had been on call the night before and was exhausted after getting very little sleep, and though I was scheduled to begin a new rotation early the next morning, I said I would without hesitation. We watched the game on the set in his hospital room, just Tom, his mother (who, truth be told, couldn't stand baseball), and me. I observed the boy as closely as I watched the television set. From the look on his face, an expression of near ecstasy, it was obvious that the boy was in heaven. "Your Yankees don't stand a chance," he told me near the end of the game, after it had become clear that the Red Sox were going to win their fifth victory in a row. ''Not a chance in the world.''

''Tom, my Yankees are still in first place by a full game,'' I pointed out, ''and there're only two games left to play. All they have to do is win both games and the Red Sox are eliminated.''

''They're going to choke,'' the boy replied. ''Believe me, this is the Sox' year. I've got a feeling.''

After the game ended I said goodbye, reminding Tom that, beginning the next morning, he'd have a new doctor. Sadly, he nodded his head; but before I left he made me promise to come back the next week and watch with him as the Sox won the American League play-off series. I told him I'd be happy to come—adding that I was sure it wouldn't be the Red Sox playing in that series, but the Yankees. I meant to keep my promise to Tom, but it proved impossible: from the beginning of my next rotation, on the infectious disease ward, I was on the go from the very first morning, with nearly no time off, bombarded both day and night by an unending parade of patients coming into the hospital with pneumonia, sepsis, and meningitis. I did manage to stop by Tom's room a few times during the second week of October. By then the boy's hair had begun to fall out, a side effect of the chemotherapy he'd been receiving, and he'd taken to wearing his Red Sox cap at all times to cover his progressive baldness. During those visits I never brought up the outcome of the pennant race, or of the play-off game that ultimately decided that contest; it had been played at Fenway Park on October 2, a game no Yankee or Red Sox fan will ever forget. In the top of the seventh inning, Bucky Dent hit a dramatic, three-run home run into the screen on top of the Green Monster, the wall in Fenway's left field, putting the Yankees ahead for good and crushing the dreams of Red Sox fans everywhere. Tom seemed depressed enough already; he was obviously severely shaken by what the chemotherapy was beginning to do to his body. Bringing up the play-off game would have been like rubbing salt into his not-yet-healed wounds.

Sometime during the middle of October, Tom, having completed his first course of chemotherapy and declared to be in remission by Kevin Donahue and the team of hematologists who were following him, was discharged from the general pediatric ward. Following his discharge, I completely lost touch with the boy.

On the first day of May, seven hard months after Tom and I had first met, I returned to the general pediatric ward for my third and final rotation. When I reported for work that morning I found that Tom Costello was a patient on the floor. I promptly barged into his room, eager to say hello. I had trouble believing what I found.

He was in a coma. Lying flat on the bed in one of the private rooms, he was unable to respond to my greeting—or, for that matter, to any other human sound. The chemotherapy he'd received since September had taken a tremendous toll on his body: he had lost all of his hair and gained at least fifty pounds, his face had become rounded and moon-shaped, and his skin had a ghostly pallor; but in spite of these side effects, the massive doses of chemotherapy had done little, if anything, to slow the progression of his cancer. "Oh, Dr. Marion, what a pleasant surprise," his mother called when she saw my face, which must have had a look of shock on it. "How nice to see you again!"

"Hello, Mrs. Costello," I replied, trying my best to regain my composure. She was sitting on an uncomfortable-looking hard-backed chair at the foot of the bed, a kindly, middle-aged Irish woman who was knitting a white sweater. "Are you working on the ward again, Dr. Marion?" she asked. I nodded and she continued: "Oh, that's grand; Tommy's wild about you. He always used to be talking about you. 'I like that Dr. Marion, even if he is a Yankees fan,' he was always telling me. He said nobody else in the hospital understood baseball the way you did."

I felt myself blush. Then, trying to give myself some

time to recover from seeing the boy and hearing his mother's words, I asked, "How's Tom been doing?"

"Not very well, I'm afraid," Mrs. Costello responded. "Dr. Donahue and the others don't hold out much hope. Still I pray, though . . ." Her voice drifted off.

I hesitated a few seconds. "Well, anything can happen, I guess," I said clumsily. "Doctors don't know everything."

"Will you be taking care of Tommy this month?" she asked, and I assured her that I would. And then, excusing myself, telling Mrs. Costello I'd return later, I went off to join the rest of the ward team for our first day of work rounds.

When we reached Tom's room on rounds that morning I asked Bill Chambers, the senior resident, if it would be okay for me to take Tom on as one of my patients. "It's fine with me," the resident replied. "Do you know his story?"

"I know he's got leukemia," I said, "and that he's on chemotherapy—"

"He does have leukemia," Bill interrupted, "but he isn't getting chemo anymore. The hematologists cut him loose."

"How come?" I asked.

"They said they've done everything they possibly can for him," Bill answered, shaking his head, "and nothing's worked. He was in remission for about four months, but then they found blast cells in his bloodstream again in January. They started him on all kinds of aggressive therapy to try to get him back into remission, but nothing's worked. The leukemic cells have taken over everything. They say his case is completely hopeless."

"There must be something they can do—some kind of therapy—"

"They say they've tried everything. They don't expect him to survive for more than another week or so. They've talked the situation over with his mother and everyone's agreed: all they want is for the kid to be kept warm, clean, and shot up with enough pain medication so he won't be uncomfortable. And that's it: no resuscitation, no heroism. You understand?'' I nodded, and we moved on to the next patient.

For the first week I went into Tom's room as infrequently as possible. Seeing the boy like that, after knowing so well how he had looked and acted at the beginning of his illness, made me incredibly sad. How little we physicians and our modern medical miracles could actually do for patients! For me, Tom was the latest in a series of children I'd cared for during the course of my internship who had withered and died before my eyes, each one demonstrating how little our ministrations mattered—how insignificant our many nights of lost sleep, our expensive and often painful diagnostic tests, our pharmacies full of medications actually proved in bringing about improvement or recovery. It seemed as if my patients either got better on their own, or they wound up like Tom Costello, waiting around to die.

It bothered me to realize how little I could help Tom. And so, to protect myself, to minimize the demoralizing damage these feelings of inadequacy could cause, I went into the boy's room only when I had to. During each visit, no matter what hour of the day or night, I found Tom and his mother in exactly the same positions they'd been in on the first day of the month; he never moved a muscle when I listened to his lungs with my stethoscope, or when I checked his pupils with my pocket flashlight. And she sat on the same hard-backed chair, busily knitting her sweater and making friendly conversation. Without saying it, she let us know by her actions that she had moved into Tom's hospital room and would be staying with the boy until the end. Every night she would drift off to sleep on that uncomfortable chair, staying close and watching as her son slowly died.

Mrs. Costello and I talked only once about baseball during the early part of that month. One day when I came in to check on the boy I noticed that standing on his bedside table was an eight-by-ten-inch framed photo-graph of Carl Yastrzemski. The picture had been auto-graphed by Yaz and carried the following message: "To Tom Costello: A hero to all of us. Get well soon!" When I asked Mrs. Costello about the photo, she told me that two months before, when Tom had still been well enough to live at home, a foundation that granted last wishes to terminally ill children had contacted the family. "Those people wanted to do something to make Tommy's last days happier," she said. "They offered a trip to Disney World, but Tommy would have none of that. He knew what he wanted from the very beginning: all he wanted was to meet Carl Yastrzemski and the rest of those Red Sox."

For the foundation, fulfilling such a wish was a cinch. They convinced the Red Sox management to hold a Tom Costello Night at Fenway Park near the beginning of the 1979 baseball season, arranging for Tom to be made hon-orary bat boy for the day and providing him with an au-thentic uniform. In all, Tom had spent six hours with the team, both in the locker room and on the field. "That night was the happiest I've ever seen him," Mrs. Cos-tello said. "And Carl Yastrzemski gave Tommy this pic-ture. It's become his most prized possession. I brought it to the hospital so that it will be the first thing he sees when he wakes up."

He went on my fourth night on call. At about nine o'clock that night Marjorie Rhodes, the evening shift nurse who had cared for the boy since the beginning of his illness, paged me. "I think Tom's about to go to heaven," she said when I returned her page from the on-call room.

"What's happening?" I asked.

"I just did his nine o'clock vital signs," she an-swered. "His pulse was down to forty and I couldn't get a blood pressure."

"I'll be right there," I said. It had been a quiet night till then, and coincidentally I had been watching the Red Sox game on the television in the on-call room. Shaking my head sadly, I turned the set off, pulled on my shoes, and headed for the ward.

They were in their usual positions. The boy's skin was paler than it had ever been, the color of fine bone china, and there was a definite tinge of blue around his lips and fingernails; his pattern of breathing was very irregular. His mother, sitting on her chair at the foot of his bed, looked up from her knitting when I entered and said, "Good evening, Dr. Marion."

"Good evening, Mrs. Costello," I replied.

"Marjorie told me that the end is near," she said, and I nodded my head. "I shouldn't be surprised," Mrs. Costello continued. "All the doctors have told me that it would end this way. Still . . ." She couldn't go on. Her eyes filled with tears.

I took my place on the right side of the boy's bed, Marjorie stood on the left, and Mrs. Costello, now putting aside her knitting, looking on from her place at the foot of the bed. And we waited for the end to come.

He lasted for another hour and a half. Slowly, Tom's breathing pattern became more and more irregular, ultimately deteriorating into what is called an agonal pattern: he would take a few deep breaths, and then all respiratory effort would cease; sixty seconds would pass, then ninety seconds, then, as I approached the bed with my stethoscope to check for a heart rate, a gasp would issue from the boy's mouth. Four or five deep breaths would follow and then the pattern would repeat itself.

As we stood at the bedside, watching and waiting, I thought back on what Tom's year had been like. He'd started it as a healthy adolescent, looking forward to the promise of a full and happy life. But then his leukemia was diagnosed. Since that time he'd been living a day-to-day existence, filled not with thoughts of the future, of high school and college, of a career and a family of his own, but rather with thoughts of white blood cell counts and too many attempts to start IVs in scarred and sclerosed veins, of bone marrow biopsies and chemotherapy protocols, of the hope of remission and the realities of the five-year survival rate. And now it was all coming to an end, all the hopes and dreams disappearing forever in a private room on the general pediatric ward at the Boston Medical Center.

When the end came at last, when two and then three minutes passed without a breath issuing from Tom's lungs, after I listened to his chest with my stethoscope and heard no sound, none of us shed a single tear. The boy's passing came as something of a relief to everyone in the room, "It's over," I said simply, and Mrs. Costello bowed her head and said a silent prayer. But she did not cry.

After allowing Mrs. Costello to be alone with Tom for a few minutes, I helped Marjorie prepare the body, and then, with her leading and me pushing the gurney, we made the long trip to the elevator at the end of the ward, down to the basement, through a tunnel, and to the holding room in the morgue that was located in the main building of the Boston Medical Center. It was eerie down in the morgue, dark and cold, and the holding room was empty except for one other body. "Thanks for coming," Marjorie said as we were making our way back toward the ward. "I usually have to make this trip by myself, and that morgue gives me the creeps!"

I nodded but remained silent. Back on the ward, we found Mrs. Costello's hard-backed chair deserted; soon after her son's death, with her work completed, the woman had quietly packed up and departed for home. I felt bad about that; I had wanted to say goodbye to her, to offer her my condolences, and I realized that now I'd probably never get the chance.

Two weeks passed. The month was coming to an end, and so, thank God, was my internship, with only one month left to go. I had been busy and pretty much put Tom and Mrs. Costello out of my mind when one morning, Ginny, the clerk on the general pediatric ward, handed me a package that had just arrived. Having never received any mail on a hospital ward before, I opened the carefully wrapped box with a great deal of curiosity. Inside, I found the sweater Mrs. Costello had been knitting, a beautiful white cardigan with the logo of the Boston Red Sox knitted over the left breast pocket. With the sweater was a note:

> Dear Dr. Marion,
>   It's been a week now since we laid Tommy to rest, but I still find it hard to believe that he is gone. The last few days have been very hard for all of us. I did not get a chance to say goodbye to you, or to thank you for the kindnesses you extended to my son on the night that he passed. Having you and Marjorie in the room with us meant more than you could ever know.
>   I hope you will accept this sweater as a token of my appreciation. I was knitting it for Tommy. I prayed that he would wear it after he made his recovery.
>
> > Sincerely yours,
> > Eileen Costello

The sweater was much too small for me, but I've kept it to this day. And whenever I think about how little I can do for my patients, or how limited medicine seems to be, I take it out of my closet and reread Mrs. Costello's note.

14

Being Right

**Eleventh month of internship,
May 1979**

"This is one of the kids I admitted yesterday," Ray East-man shouted as the general pediatric ward team gathered around him in the infants' room. Our team had just begun its usual morning work rounds and Ray, the intern who had been on call the night before, was trying his best to give us a rundown on all the patients he had admitted during the previous twenty-four hours. But the child whose history he was attempting to report, a small infant who had been placed in one of the four steel-barred cribs that filled the small room to capacity, was at that moment screaming so loudly that all of us were having trouble hearing anything Ray said. To compensate, the intern had turned up his volume: "His name's Brian McCallister," Ray continued, "and his pediatrician was concerned because he wasn't gaining enough weight, so he sent him in to the GI clinic. Dr. Rogers saw Brian yesterday and was so impressed by his puniness that he immediately decided to admit the kid for a million-dollar workup."

"How old's this kid?" Bill Chambers, the senior resident in charge of our team that month, asked the intern, also shouting his question over the baby's hoarse cry.

167

"He'll be exactly a year old next week," Ray answered.

"He *is* pretty small," said Jennifer Kaplan, the third intern on our team, while trying to force a pacifier into the baby's mouth to get the kid to shut up. "He looks about right for a four-month-old." But little Brian wouldn't have any of that pacifier; he just spat the rubber nipple out and kept on screaming. "And he seems pretty irritable, too."

"Irritable is an understatement," I said.

"Is he always like this," Bill asked, "or is this a manifestation of some recently acquired, horrible new disease?"

"Nah," Ray hollered back. "I don't think he's got any new disease; his mother told me he's always been in excellent health. And I don't think he's usually this pissed off, either; I think he's probably just angry because his mother's not around. She told me she's also got a three-year-old at home to take care of. She said she'd come back sometime later today if she could get someone to watch the other kid."

"Did she give you any idea of what she thought might be wrong with this one?" Bill asked. "Is his problem that he doesn't eat, or does he eat and just not grow?"

"She told me that Brian never seems to be hungry," the intern replied. "She said that since she brought him home from the hospital after he was first born she's nearly had to force-feed him in order to get him to take anything. She described him as a fretful eater, whatever the hell that means."

"I think it means that he screams at the top of his lungs whenever anyone gets near him," Jennifer said. "He sure is puny! Look at those arms and legs; they're like toothpicks. And his face looks kind of funny, too, doesn't it?"

Standing at Jennifer's side and listening to the conversation, I too had noticed that this baby looked a little unusual. Staring down at the child, who was lying on the crib's mattress with his eyes closed, his mouth open, and his face bright red from the bout of screaming in which he was then involved, I had the strange feeling that I'd seen this infant someplace. I couldn't put my finger on where, though. "Has he ever been in this hospital before?" I shouted in the general direction of Ray.

"No," he said. "Before yesterday, he's never been anywhere around here."

"He does look kind of funny," Bill agreed. "Did you find anything unusual when you examined him?"

"Nope. Outside of the fact that he's so small and, like you guys said, that he looks kind of funny, he seemed perfectly fine to me. I spent a long time looking at his face last night when I was trying to get some blood out of him; his veins are as scrawny as the rest of him, so I had a lot of opportunity to study him. And you know what? All at once it hit me: doesn't this kid look like a gnome?"

Bill and Jennifer both began to laugh, and the resident shouted, "Now that you mention it, he does look kind of gnomelike. You put him in one of those pointy little red hats, and he'd be all set." But I didn't laugh along with the rest of the team because just then a distant bell began to ring in my head, a bell that had remained deathly silent during the previous eleven months of my internship, a sound that represented unconnected, scattered thoughts beginning to come together in my brain. At that moment I realized where I'd seen this child's face before: it had been in one of my favorite books, a text by David Smith, M.D., entitled *Recognizable Patterns of Human Malformations*, a volume composed of pictures of infants and children with unusual and rare genetic disorders, a book I'd kept by my bedside and studied at odd moments since I'd been a third-year medical student and had nearly committed to memory. "This kid's not a gnome," I blurted out. "He's an elf! He's got Williams syndrome!"

The other members of the team stopped laughing and looked up at me as if I was crazy, but the longer I stared at the baby the more convinced I became that Brian did, in fact, have Williams syndrome, a rare disorder that, among other problems, causes growth retardation, poor feeding, and during infancy, irritability. "I'll prove it," I yelled over Brian's crying. "Stay right here." And without another word I rushed down the hallway of the general pediatric ward, away from the screaming of the infant, and out into the tiny room that doubled as our intern on-call room and house-staff library. Excitedly, I began searching the shelves for a copy of the book. . . .

The Wednesday on which Ray Eastman presented the case of Brian McCallister to our team marked something of a milestone in my career as an intern. On that morning, for the first time since the year began, I awakened knowing I was going to survive internship. For months before, I had seriously wondered whether I'd be able to make it through the whole year; but when, on that morning in late May, during my ritual of lying in bed and counting the number of nights on call I had left until the new interns were scheduled to arrive during the last days of June, I realized that the magic number had dwindled to ten—to a quantity that, literally, I could count on the fingers of my two hands—I broke into a grin from ear to ear. Soon my internship would be a thing of the past.

Although this realization succeeded in clearing many of my concerns out of my head, it also led to a new fear. For a full year I had functioned as an automaton: I'd spent my days, as well as my nights on call, performing jobs that other people ordered me to perform; down to the smallest detail, my work time was planned out for me by others, residents, fellows, and attending physicians, who led me by the hand, like a child, through the management of every patient for whom I was responsible, telling me exactly what I had to do and precisely when I had to do it. During the entire year I had been permitted to develop and act on virtually no spontaneous, creative thought. On the very few occasions I tried to offer an opinion about a patient based on an original idea I was shot down by my superiors, told that interns were paid to work, not to think. I was so used to this treatment that, now that the year was finally coming to an end, I was beginning to doubt whether I'd ever be able to think on my own again.

That, I guess, was the reason why, on that Wednesday morning on the general pediatric ward, it suddenly became so important to me to prove to the senior resident and my fellow interns that this irritable baby who had been admitted to the general pediatric ward for a workup of his failure to thrive had this rare disorder known as Williams syndrome. I needed to prove to myself that, thinking on my own, I was still capable of making a diagnosis.

At that time I had never actually seen a patient with Williams syndrome, but I thought I knew everything there was to know about the disease. During medical school, for some strange reason that still isn't clear to me, I had become interested in multiple malformation syndromes, patterns of congenital defects that tend to cluster together in unrelated children. David Smith's book of syndromes played a key role in fostering this weird interest. I spent hours pouring over the second edition of the book whenever I had a spare moment, gazing at the pictures of affected patients and reading the descriptions that accompanied them, until I seemed to have learned it all. On that morning all those hours of studying paid off: I knew all about Williams syndrome, and I was certain that Brian McCallister had it.

Finding the book on the third shelf of the house-staff library, I pulled the volume out and ran with it back up to the ward, to the infants' room. On my return, Brian seemed a bit calmer: he was still making some noise, but he wasn't screaming as loudly as he had been before. The team hadn't waited for me; in the relative quiet they'd moved on to other patients, and at the moment of my return Ray was discussing another of his admissions from the night before, a baby with diarrhea and dehydration who had been placed in the crib next to Brian's. But I insisted that the team return to Brian's bedside and stare down at his face again.

"I'm right about this, I know it," I exclaimed, opening Smith's text to the pictures and descriptions of Williams syndrome. Holding the book close to Brian's face, I said, "See? Flaring of the eyebrows, small, bright blue eyes with puffiness around them, depressed nasal bridge, prominent lips and ears, short stature; this kid's got everything listed in the book! He's got it; I'm positive!"

"Hang on a minute, Bob," Bill replied. "You might be right about this, but as I recall, kids with Williams syndrome have all sorts of other problems, don't they? Don't they have mental retardation and heart disease—"

"He did have a slight heart murmur," Ray interrupted. "I guess I forgot to mention that."

"Yeah, well, a slight heart murmur isn't enough," Bill continued. "These kids have something weird, don't they?"

"Supravalvular aortic stenosis," I said, reading from the book. I had no idea what supravalvular aortic stenosis was, other than that it was a congenital defect of the heart.

"Right," Bill continued. "And don't they have some metabolic problem, like elevated levels of calcium in their blood?"

"Yeah," I replied, again looking at the book. "It says hypercalcemia is an occasional abnormality."

"We don't know if he's got any of that stuff," Bill said. He was silent for a few seconds. "Do you know how rare this syndrome is?" the senior resident finally asked.

"But kids with Williams syndrome do have poor growth," Jennifer pointed out.

"And Brian does look like the pictures in the book," Ray added.

"You guys think Bob might be right about this?" Bill asked.

"Nobody else has come up with a suggestion that makes any more sense," Jennifer said.

Again Bill hesitated. "Well, I'm sure they're going to wind up doing just about every test in the book on this kid, anyway," the resident concluded. "I guess it wouldn't hurt to work him up for Williams syndrome while we're at it. What do you think we should do?''

"A cardiologist should see him," Ray began, "to check if he's got that supravalvular aortic stenosis. He'll probably need to have an echocardiogram to prove it.''

"And we should probably get a calcium level," Jennifer continued.

"That's good for a start," Bill said. "And we ought to have the geneticists come over and check him out. But see if you can get Dr. Bloomenfeld himself to come rather than one of his fellows; Oscar knows more about syndromes than just about anybody else in the world.''

"I'll take care of it," Ray replied, writing the plans down on his clipboard. And then we moved on to the next patient.

Oscar Bloomenfeld showed up early that afternoon. The director of the clinical genetics service and a professor of pediatrics at the Boston Medical Center, Dr. Bloomenfeld was nationally known for his work in the field of dysmorphology, the study of birth defects and how they assemble themselves into syndromes, sharing the spotlight with my personal hero, David Smith, the man who had written the book *Recognizable Patterns of Human Malformations*. His role as medical correspondent also made him a local television celebrity, appearing on the six and eleven o'clock newscasts nearly every night.

It was a little unusual for Dr. Bloomenfeld to make a personal appearance on the general pediatric ward. Most of the time, when an opinion about a patient was required, Dr. Bloomenfeld would send one of his postdoctoral fellows to do the work. But when Ray called the genetics office that morning to request a consultation, he asked specifically for the boss, and surprisingly, Oscar Bloomenfeld honored the request. And so, when we saw the big man walk through the doors at the entrance to the ward, Ray, Jennifer and I, each trying to get our morning scut work finished, stopped what we were doing and followed the professor into the infants' room. On my way into the room I didn't exactly walk; I kind of strutted. Positive that Bloomenfeld would take one look at Brian, agree with me immediately, and offer me a job as his associate when I completed my training, I was unable to conceal the pride I felt for having first made the diagnosis of this rare disorder.

But agree with my impression was not exactly what Oscar Bloomenfeld did. He walked to the crib, took one look at the infant, and frowned. Turning toward us, he said to Ray, "You're Eastman, right?" Ray nodded, and the attending continued: "You're pulling my leg, aren't you, Eastman? You don't really believe this kid's got Williams, do you?"

"Well . . ." Ray began, pointing in my direction. "That is, Bob here . . ."

Dr. Bloomenfeld now looked toward me. "You're Marion, right? The one who wants to be a geneticist when he grows up?"

I nodded meekly, my cockiness gone, and I suddenly wished I could crawl under a baseboard. "You really think this kid's got Williams?" the attending asked.

I half-nodded this time, losing my self-confidence as Dr. Bloomenfeld continued: "You've got to be crazy. This kid doesn't look anything like a Williams. He is small and he may have something, but it sure as hell isn't Williams syndrome."

"You don't think that's an elfinlike facial appearance?" I asked submissively.

"Marion," he said in reply, "I'm so sure he doesn't have Williams syndrome that I'm willing to bet on it. You guys sent off a calcium level already, didn't you?" All three of us nodded now. "Okay, then; I'll bet you a nickel the calcium level comes back completely normal. And I'll bet you another nickel that the cardiologists don't find anything wrong with this kid's heart, especially not supravalvular aortic stenosis. Want to take me up on it?"

I felt like an idiot, but something told me I was right about Brian's diagnosis. So I told the internationally known geneticist and television personality that yes, I would take him up on his bets, and we shook hands. As he left the floor Dr. Bloomenfeld, grinning, said, "It's a good thing we have you interns around. You suckers haven't figured out yet that I only bet on sure things."

At seven o'clock I was home, engaged in what had become my usual off-call evening routine: I was lying in bed naked, watching reruns of old situation comedies on WSBK, one of the local UHF television stations, while eating a greasy pizza I had picked up on the way home from work at the Watertown Pizza House. My mind wasn't on that night's episode of "The Odd Couple," though. I had been thinking about Oscar Bloomenfeld and his response to Brian McCallister's physical appearance most of the day, and my replay of the events intensified during this television hour. I was shaken by what had happened, but I still had the feeling that I was right.

During my fourth year of medical school I had learned not to be overly eager to offer my opinions regarding patients' diagnoses. But Brian McCallister's case was different: even after Oscar Bloomenfeld had written his note in the chart and left the floor, I simply hadn't been convinced that I was wrong; even after I had looked at the note and read the master geneticist's opinion that no evidence existed for the child's having Williams or any other syndrome, I had a great deal of confidence in my diagnosis.

I was fighting my way through the pizza when the telephone rang. A very excited-sounding Jennifer Kaplan was on the other end of the receiver. "Bob, you're not going to believe this," she said. "The cardiologist just finished doing an echocardiogram on Brian McCallister. Guess what he found!"

"Supravalvular aortic stenosis," I said as casually as possible, even though I was almost choking on a glob of mozzarrella cheese. "What else?"

"Correct," she replied.

"Did his calcium level come back from the lab?"

"Yeah," she answered, "about an hour ago. It was ten-point-seven; the upper limit of normal is ten-five. You were right, Bob; the kid absolutely does have Williams syndrome! You were right, and the world-famous Dr. Oscar Bloomenfeld was wrong!"

"Amazing!" I said, grinning broadly.

Jennifer had a lot of work to do, so we hung up and I returned to my pizza in celebration. As I chewed happily I became as pumped up as a blowfish; the laboratory data had proven the lowly intern correct and the nationally known geneticist dead wrong. I was thinking of looking up Oscar's home number in the telephone book so I could call and tell him the news personally that night. I was exuberant.

My exultation lasted as long as the pizza held out.

By then "The Odd Couple" ended and my thoughts shifted from my extraordinary clinical acumen to the fact that Brian McCallister actually had Williams syndrome. And all at once I realized that something was very wrong. I had become overjoyed to have been correct in making a diagnosis, a diagnosis that was at that moment adversely affecting an infant. I had predicted that the child had a disease that was chronic and potentially life-shortening and that, at the very least, would disrupt his family and leave the child mildly to moderately retarded and abnormally small. At the worst, it would cause him to have severe heart problems that could require risky cardiac surgery followed by a long period of recuperation and years and years of follow-up visits with the cardiologist. Was it possible that I could actually have become exuberant about such a thing? What had happened to me, the guy whose motivation for becoming a doctor in the first place had been to find some way to help his fellow man?

Beth came into the bedroom soon after and we turned out the lights, but I had a lot of trouble falling asleep that night, an occurrence that is more than a little rare in the life of a chronically overtired intern. As I lay awake in bed, I kept turning this seeming paradox over in my mind. At about two o'clock in the morning, I was able to hold it in no longer; I switched on the light and awakened Beth.

"What do you want from me?" she asked, as I nudged her out of her sound sleep and back to consciousness.

"I've got this problem, Beth—" I began.

"What . . . what's wrong?" she interrupted, coming to attention.

"You know that kid I told you about, the one who seems to have Williams syndrome?"

"Yeah," Beth asked, yawning. "You were right and that famous TV doctor was wrong. You should be proud of yourself. What about it?"

"That's what the problem is," I answered. "See, I'm actually happy that the kid's got Williams syndrome. What right do I have to feel happy about it when this kid's going to lead such a lousy life?"

Beth was silent for a few seconds. "You woke me up to ask me a question like that?" she finally asked.

"Yeah," I said. "It's really bothering me."

"You're feeling guilty because you were the only person who made the right diagnosis?"

"Not that I made the diagnosis," I replied. "I feel guilty because I'm happy and excited about it."

"Boy, has this year screwed you up!" my wife said. "Bob, you're not happy and excited because the kid's got that syndrome; you're happy and excited because you made a diagnosis that the world-famous hot-shot geneticist couldn't make. That means you're a good doctor and that you're on the ball. The fact that you made the diagnosis doesn't have anything to do with the fact that the kid's got this weird disease; he would have had it whether or not you or anyone else had thought of it. He would've wound up being just as retarded, and having just as much heart disease. Don't you see that?"

I was silent for a few seconds. "I guess."

"Bob, think about it for a minute: you did this kid and his family a lot of good. If you hadn't thought of the diagnosis today, what would have happened?"

"The kid would've had a million-dollar workup," I said after a few seconds' pause.

"Right," Beth continued. "And what would that million-dollar workup have shown?"

"I guess that the kid had supravalvular aortic stenosis and hypercalcemia," I concluded.

"That's right. Somebody would have ultimately made a diagnosis of this Williams syndrome anyway. What you did by making the diagnosis was save the kid from having to go through all those stupid, worthless tests that would have been normal."

Again I was silent. "I guess you have a point," I said. "But still, it doesn't feel right—"

"I don't give a damn about how it feels," Beth interrupted. "That's just the way it is. Now if it's all right with you, I'd like to try to get back to Dreamland."

That ended our conversation; no longer bothered by a nagging, half-crazed husband, Beth fell right back into a sound sleep; but I stayed awake the rest of the night. Unfortunately, I've never completely resolved the seeming paradox I uncovered that day. Even today, in my role as clinical geneticist, when I make a diagnosis that carries a bad prognosis, I think back to that baby with Williams syndrome and feel that emotional tugging in two separate directions.

Ten years after finishing my internship I was sitting in my office at the Center for Congenital Disorders at the hospital at which I work in the Bronx, counseling a couple whose sixteen-month-old son, Jonathan Mason, had just been diagnosed as having Williams syndrome. The child, who, like Brian McCallister, had been cranky and irritable during much of his infancy but had now developed the outgoing, loquacious personality that for some reason occurs in toddlers with this disorder, had been referred to me by a friend of the family's. I had made the diagnosis on first laying eyes on Jonathan, while he and his parents were still seated in the waiting room. I sent them to a cardiologist who, on the basis of an echocardiogram, had diagnosed mild supravalvular aortic stenosis, thus confirming the diagnosis.

"Why didn't any of the other doctors pick this up?" Mr. Mason asked, skeptical of my diagnosis. Before coming to see me, the Masons had taken Jonathan to see more than a dozen physicians in the New York metropolitan area, top specialists in gastroenterology, child development, cardiology, and general pediatrics. These physicians had offered special diets for the child in an attempt to get him to grow, prescribed physical and occupational therapy to get his delayed development back on track, and even offered vitamins and other medications. But apparently no one had seen what I'd seen, and none of the treatments that had been offered had done the child the least bit of good. "He saw so many experts and went through so many tests, it's hard to believe that not one other person came up with this diagnosis."

"Williams syndrome isn't very common," I explained. "It's not something physicians see every day. Unfortunately, this kind of story, of a child with Williams syndrome being seen by lots of specialists before the right diagnosis is made, is pretty common. I guess I've become something of a specialist in Williams syndrome and that's really how I knew that Jonathan had this condition the moment I first saw him."

What I told Mr. Mason was completely true. Whether because of the involvement with Brian McCallister late in my internship or whether because of a deep interest I'd always had in this disorder is not clear, but over the years, during the course of my training and later as a practicing clinical geneticist, I had become something of an expert in the area of the diagnosis and treatment of children with Williams syndrome. I'd published articles and abstracts on the natural history of the condition in the medical literature, testified as an expert witness about the disorder at a malpractice trial, and diagnosed over twenty children like Jonathan, counseling their parents about the consequences of this rare disease, helping to guide their medical, and when necessary, surgical management, and watching them slowly grow and develop at their individual pace.

"And his personality, his eyes—everything—you think are the result of this—this Williams syndrome?" Mrs. Mason asked, sounding even more skeptical than her husband.

"I'm sure of it." I took out my office copy of David Smith's book, then in its fourth edition, and showed them the pictures and description of the syndrome. The couple studied the pages carefully and silently. "It's amazing," the father finally said, the doubt completely gone from his voice. "That's Jonathan all right. That's Jon to a tee!"

Now that they were convinced, I sat and spoke with Mr. and Mrs. Mason for over an hour. As Jonathan played on the floor of my office, I explained the disorder to them as best I could; I counseled them about the genetic risk of recurrence in subsequent children; I told them what the future might hold for Jonathan and for them. During our conversation the Masons gained a good deal of information, and I felt I'd acquired a fair amount of insight about them.

Near the end of our meeting Jonathan began to fuss, and his father excused himself and went out to the waiting room to get the child's bottle. He returned to my office with a puzzled look on his face. "You said this was a rare disease, didn't you, Dr. Marion?" Mr. Mason asked as he returned to his seat.

"Yes," I replied. "It occurs in about one in twenty thousand newborns. What makes you ask?"

"Well, I just saw the patient who's sitting out in the waiting room," the father answered, "and it looks like she's got Williams syndrome, too."

"No, I don't think so," I replied, smiling. "As far as I know, there are no other patients with Williams syndrome scheduled to be seen today."

"Well, there's a kid out there who could be Jonathan's twin. It's eerie. If my son's got Williams syndrome, that kid's got it, too."

I shrugged my shoulders, not wanting to get into an argument about the vagaries of syndrome identification with this man. I changed the subject. Within another few minutes, we were finished. While shaking hands with the couple, I told them not to hesitate to call if they had any questions in the future.

Holding Jonathan in my arms, I was walking the Masons out to the secretary's desk in order to schedule a follow-up appointment for six months when I saw her: my next patient, a thirteen-month-old girl who had been referred for evaluation of failure to thrive and developmental delay. At the sight of that little girl, my mouth dropped open and I was rendered unable to utter a sound. It was immediately clear to me, as it had been to Jonathan Mason's father, that this little girl did indeed have Williams syndrome.

I guess my amazement at seeing that little girl had two separate components. First, I was startled at the coincidence, the twist of secretarial fate that allowed these two children, whose very rare congenital malformation syndrome had gone undiagnosed for the first year of their lives, to be scheduled for back-to-back appointments on the same afternoon. The odds against something like that happening had to be astronomical.

But more than that, I was stunned that Jonathan Mason's father was able to make the correct diagnosis of this unusual disorder, a diagnosis that, as was the case with his own son, had been missed by doctor after doctor, after gazing at that little girl for no more than thirty seconds. Perhaps I shouldn't have been so amazed by this fact, though: after all, if an intern with nearly no experience could be right about the diagnosis of Williams syndrome when the famous dysmorphologist Oscar Bloomenfeld had been wrong, nearly anything could happen.

The end came without any fanfare. On June 27, 1979, for the last time in my internship, I signed out my patients and was free. Although I had a lot to do in order to get ready for our return to New York, there was still a little time left for some celebrating.

15

Checking Out

**Last day of internship,
June 27, 1979**

The bar was cool and dark and almost empty as I sat on a stool, sipping my beer. The peace and quiet were exactly what I needed, a luxury that I'd more than earned; for a few minutes at least I had absolutely nothing else to do, nothing other than sit and reflect on the experience that was now finished. I had been waiting for this day to come for a whole year, and now it was here. At long last, I'd reached the final day of my internship.

I had been on call the night before and, as usual, hadn't gotten much sleep, but was wide awake and at full attention when the new interns began to arrive in the lobby of the pediatric wing at a little before eight that morning. I watched them assemble in the main conference room to begin their day of orientation, their eyes wide as saucers, their hands trembling slightly. Had I looked that scared when I reported for work exactly one year before? I didn't think so; I didn't remember being frightened. Of course, anything was possible: after all, I could barely remember things that had happened the previous week. I felt sorry for these new interns, these poor little lambs; they didn't have a clue concerning the horrors that were about to befall them.

But I wasn't able to consider the plight of the new

interns for very long; I had a tremendous amount of work to get done that day. Exactly one year before, during our orientation session, representatives from all the hospital's administrative services had come, parading themselves in front of the fourteen of us new interns in that same conference room. The program had been well organized: while sitting in that room we were issued parking cards, white doctor's coats and pants, and beepers; documents were brought to us, and we all silently filled out our health records and our contracts, our Drug Enforcement Agency forms and our vow to uphold the rules of the medical center. But checking out of internship was far from organized: the process was a complicated, seemingly unending scavenger hunt. In order to gain my freedom, it would be necessary for me to tour the entire Boston Medical Center, dropping off some item here, signing some document there, making sure to get a key person's initials on something called the Master Internship Release Form at each stop along the way. The whole thing was a huge pain in the ass, but the prize at the end of the hunt, when all the junk was back where it belonged, all the forms had been signed, and all the initials had been collected, was release from the bondage of internship.

So, with more energy than I ever remembered having after a night on call, I wrote off-service notes in the charts of all my patients, signed out to the poor intern who was unfortunate enough to draw call on the very last night of the year, and began the process of getting my Master Internship Release Form completed. And with each stop along the way, a memory or two would come into my mind. . . .

I started in the parking garage. I was more than happy to surrender my parking card, which hadn't been used since a very bad Friday night back in early February.

It had been the end of a horrible week, a week that began with a Sunday on call in the emergency room. We were at the tail end of flu season, and I had spent most of the night seeing the patients who had registered at the triage desk. We changed services the next morning, and I moved on to begin my second month of work on the general pediatric ward. Bleary-eyed, I spent the entire day, while fighting desperately to stay awake, trying to figure out what the hell was going on with the dozen or so patients I had inherited from the interns who had worked there the month before.

Because of the change of service, I'd pulled what we called an every-other, being scheduled for call again on Tuesday night. That had been another tough night, and I was looking forward to a couple of days without call following it, but then, when I showed up for work Thursday morning, I found that the intern who was supposed to be working that night had developed gastroenteritis, becoming so sick that she was at that moment lying in the emergency room with an intravenous line stuck into her arm. "I know you've just come off an every-other," said Dan, our chief resident, when he talked to me before work rounds got under way that morning, "but you're going to have to work again tonight. I have nobody else to cover the ward." I didn't say a word in protest; I had come to understand that arguing about such things would get me nowhere. So I simply nodded and made plans to stay the night.

But the week was at last behind me, and as I headed out to my car that Friday night, I held my head high: I'd spent over 110 hours in the hospital over the previous six days, and I knew that if I could survive that, I could survive anything.

As I started up my car that evening, I thought about how things had changed. The whole internship seemed to have come together over the course of the previous few weeks. A month before I had been very insecure; I'd still had some trouble drawing blood and starting IVs, and I had virtually no clinical judgment whatsoever. But during that week, it seemed as if I'd turned into the consummate intern, suddenly becoming reliable, responsible, and technically adept (in other words, an automaton).

As I left the parking garage and pulled out into the darkened streets of Boston I realized that, from here on, the rest of the year should be a cinch.

In fact, during the first part of that drive I wasn't even tired. As the car headed onto the traffic-choked Massachusetts Turnpike I decided that, in honor of my new-found medical competence, I would take Beth out for dinner at a new Chinese restaurant we'd both been wanting to try in Cambridge. And after dinner we could try to catch a movie at the Orson Welles Cinema; or maybe we'd even drive up the coast to Rockport to watch the sunrise in the morning. Hell, I was feeling so good, I figured I could do anything.

The traffic was only creeping along; for some reason, the Pike that night was much more congested than usual. A J. Geils song came on on the radio; I cranked up the volume and sang along at the top of my voice. But then as the song ended and the news came on, my mind kind of drifted off. . . .

A man was shaking me vigorously by the shoulders. I heard sirens off in the distance, and the guy was saying, "Hey, wake up. Are you all right? Are you asleep?"

"What . . . what happened?" I asked groggily. The man explained that I'd just driven my car directly into a concrete retaining wall.

The cops arrived a few minutes later. It was fortunate that there was so much traffic that night. Had I been going any faster than five or ten miles an hour, I probably would have hit that retaining wall with enough force to total the car and kill myself. As it was, I was fine, and the car's right front fender would only need a few hundred dollars' worth of body work. But that was enough for me: I accepted the warning I'd been given without hesitation.

Beth and I didn't get to see the sunrise over Rockport the next morning, or on any other morning during my internship year. We never made it to the Orson Welles Cinema that night, and I didn't even eat dinner. With a final burst of adrenaline surging through my body, I managed to drive the crippled car home without further incident. I barely made it onto our living room couch before the adrenaline high finally gave out.

Somehow Beth got me off the couch and into bed, where I slept soundly for the next sixteen hours. And when I finally awoke and explained to her what had happened to the car, she reached into my pants pocket, removed my key chain, and stripped me of my car keys. "I agreed to be a widow to this internship for one year," she told me, "but I refuse to allow you to commit suicide with a moving vehicle. From now on, you're taking the bus."

And so it was. For the remainder of the year I left the driving to the professionals of the Metropolitan Boston Transit Authority. The bus, which left from Watertown Square, let me off a few blocks from the medical center. That twice-daily walk, to and from the bus stop, was the only exercise I got during the remainder of my internship year, and more important, the MBTA drivers managed to keep me alive and safe from Boston traffic (and vice versa).

On that Friday night in early February I learned two important lessons: first, if I don't get at least six hours of sleep a week, I become completely incoherent; and second, interns make terrible drivers.

After getting my Master Internship Release Form initialed by the director of the parking garage, I proceeded on to the laundry room, where, in exchange for the laundry director's initials, I surrendered the four pairs of spotlessly clean white pants and doctor's coats I'd received during orientation. Because interns in pediatrics were not required to wear whites to work, these articles had hung, undisturbed, in my closet since that day.

From the laundry I headed to the employees' health service clinic, where I had to undress and undergo a complete physical exam. The health service doctor poked and prodded me; he measured my weight, pulse rate, and blood pressure; with his stethoscope, he listened to my heart and lungs; he palpated my abdomen and pounded the area of my back lying over my kidneys. And when he had finished, he told me that I was in excellent health. This news didn't surprise me: during the previous year, I'd learned how very little physical examinations and laboratory tests actually tell about a patient's condition, and this examination proved the point. I wasn't in excellent health that day; I wasn't even in good health. I was fat, having gained over fifteen pounds during the time I'd been in Boston. I was out of shape, since I hadn't had time for exercise, other than my walks between the bus stop and the medical center, for the entire previous year. I was chronically overtired, overstressed, and overburdened, and my spirit and my heart had been broken. But none of this was uncovered in the physical exam the health service doctor performed. And so, like the others, he too initialed my form.

I spent the next hour visiting various administrative offices: medical records, where, miraculously, I'd been listed as having successfully completed all of my patients' charts; payroll, which I informed of the new address in the Bronx where my remaining paychecks should be forwarded; and then on to the medical center post office, where I cleared out all the junk mail that had accumulated in my box over the past couple of months, tossing it directly into the trash, and handed in my key.

Having saved the best for last, I then moved on to the final stop, winding up my tour that afternoon in the communications office, the place on the top floor of the main building of the Boston Medical Center from which my beeper had been controlled. The calm, grandmotherly women who inhabited the office were the page operators who had run my life during the previous twelve months. But they would control me no longer: as I removed the small silver box from the place on my belt where it had hung for the last year and handed it over to the director of the office, I breathed a sigh of relief. But before I could relax, before I was completely home free, a snag developed: studying my beeper closely, the director got a confused look on her face. "There seems to be something wrong here, Dr. Marion," she said. "I have you listed as having received beeper one forty-seven, not two twenty-six. How did you get this other beeper?" And so, before leaving, I had to tell her the story of Christina Castellano and her older brother, Jeremy.

Christina was one of the patients I had inherited when I'd begun working in the neonatal intensive care unit at the start of my second month of internship. Born by cesarean section at South Shore Hospital, a community hospital in the suburbs of Boston, the child had been in excellent health until her sixth day of life, just before she was scheduled to be discharged from the hospital, when she developed a mild case of diarrhea. As a result of the diarrhea, the doctors decided to keep Christina in the hospital for a few extra days; they also changed her formula from Similac, which contained cow's milk, to Prosobee, which was soybean-based. Christina's diarrhea resolved over the next few days, but the infant became lethargic and began to feed poorly. Fearing that the child might be suffering from some rare inborn error of metabolism, a defect in the way her body broke down the food it received, her pediatrician arranged an immediate transfer to the Boston Medical Center for further evaluation.

At first it seemed that the pediatrician had been correct: initial laboratory tests performed on Christina at the medical center in fact revealed a very unusual metabolic disturbance. The experts who were called on to offer opinions about what was causing the child's problem at the start of her hospitalization were baffled by the abnormalities that had been detected. No one had ever seen a child quite like Christina, and as a result, a million-dollar workup was undertaken.

But during the first few days after her admission to our hospital, something amazing happened: Christina's lethargy lifted and she began eating and acting more like a normal child. Paralleling these changes in her clinical condition, the infant's previously out-of-whack laboratory parameters all spontaneously returned to normal. Not surprisingly, the expensive and exotic laboratory tests that had been performed failed to reveal any obvious underlying abnormality. Nearly everyone in the hospital remained completely confused about the patient's disease as well as by its sudden resolution.

One person did, however, suggest a plausible explanation. Early on during Christina Castellano's hospital stay, Miriam Doyle, the hospital's nutritionist, postulated that the metabolic disturbances seen in the child's initial blood tests could all be explained by the method used to mix up the formula the child had been receiving while at South Shore Hospital. The symptoms Christina had suffered, and the laboratory abnormalities accompanying those symptoms, were observed only after the child had been switched to Prosobee at South Shore; furthermore, these aberrations had rapidly cleared up once the formula was discontinued. Miriam at once phoned the pharmaceutical company that made Prosobee and asked that the batch of formula from which South Shore Hospital's supply had originated be checked. The manufacturer's response came the day after I arrived in the NICU, and it proved that the nutritionist's hunch was correct.

Miriam and I invited Christina's parents into the small conference room of the neonatal intensive care unit to discuss the results of the company's investigation. Because they hadn't been able to get a baby-sitter that afternoon, Mr. and Mrs. Castellano had brought their other child, seven-year-old Jeremy, to the hospital with them; out of necessity, Jeremy had to join us in the conference room.

I was a little reluctant to allow Jeremy into the room. The boy had spent a good deal of time around the hospital during the two and a half weeks Christina had been there, and I'd already heard a half-dozen horror stories about the kid, who was extremely hyperactive and who, according to Norma Kennedy, the intern who had been

in charge of Christina's case before I started in the NICU,
had "very poor impulse control."

Norma told me the following story: on the day after
Christina's admission to the NICU, she had done a lumbar puncture on the infant because one of the neurologists wanted to get his hands on some of the child's
priceless spinal fluid. It had been a difficult spinal tap,
taking Norma nearly an hour to complete. She drained
out just enough fluid to satisfy the neurologist, and before going off to fill out the necessary lab slips she left
the precious, carefully capped plastic tube at the side of
the infant's crib for safekeeping. When Norma returned
to Christina's bedside, she found the critical tube in Jeremy's hot little hands; the cap was open and the tube
emptied. "What did you do with that fluid?" Mrs. Castellano asked her son. The boy responded by pointing to
his mouth and patting his belly. "You drank it?" Mrs.
Castellano asked, and the boy nodded angelically. The
things Norma mumbled under her breath as she carried
Christina back into the treatment room to repeat the spinal tap, however, were apparently far from angelic.

Although Miriam and I would rather have talked with
the parents without Jeremy in the room, we had no
choice: no one willing to watch the boy was available.
And so we entered that little conference room together.

The place was stifling. Boston was in the midst of a
heat wave and the hospital was not air-conditioned. While
the Castellanos took seats at the conference table, I threw
open the room's only window. "We've got some great
news," Miriam Doyle began. "The company that makes
Prosobee finally called me back this morning. Apparently there was a problem with the formula Christina received at South Shore Hospital. Somehow, four times the
normal amount of salt got added to the vat, and it threw
off your baby's electrolyte balance."

"You mean there's nothing wrong with Christina?"
Mr. Castellano asked. At this point Jeremy, who had been
sitting on his mother's lap, started to get bored. He stood

up and began marching around the conference room like a soldier.

"Nothing that caused this particular problem," I answered, trying to ignore the boy, who had picked up a few pieces of chalk from the blackboard and was just then shoving them into his mouth.

"Get that chalk out of your mouth this second!" Mrs. Castellano shouted at her son. After flashing one of those angelic looks toward his mother, Jeremy spat the entire wad of saliva-soaked chalk pieces across the room, narrowly missing his mother's left ear. "So you were right all along," the mother said to Miriam, after flashing an angry look toward her son. "You were right and the doctors were wrong. What a relief!"

"You can say that again," Mr. Castellano added. "Is there a chance that Christina might have suffered any permanent damage as a result of this?" While his father was speaking Jeremy, with no more chalk pieces to keep him busy, had found a stack of paper which had been left at the head of the conference table; the boy began tossing the papers, one by one, into the air.

"Jeremy, stop that right now!" Mrs. Castellano ordered, and once again he complied with her request.

"We can't be completely sure," Miriam replied to Mr. Castellano's question, "but all the specialists around here think that she'll be fine."

"We'll have to keep an eye on her in the future," I added, "looking for some of the problems that are known to occur in children who have had severe electrolyte imbalances during the newborn period." Suddenly, the lights in the conference room began switching on and off.

"Jeremy, stop that immediately!" Mr. Castellano said, but the boy didn't cease his flashing of the lights until his mother hollered at him to come and sit down. Dutifully, he did so, without hesitation.

"What kind of problems would you be worried about?" Mr. Castellano asked.

"Things like delay in development, or seizures, or learning disabilities," I responded. "It's not that we expect any of these things to happen; it's just that those are the kinds of problems that sometimes occur.''

''Oh, I pray that's not the case,'' Mrs. Castellano said. ''I don't know what we'd do if Christina turns out to be like Jeremy. There's no way we'd be able to handle two kids like this!''

''He does seem like a handful,'' I replied. Although he was still sitting next to his mother, Jeremy had begun kicking his feet against the legs of the conference room table. The table, which was old and rickety, jumped an inch or two into the air with every blow, and I was positive the thing was about to collapse. ''Does he go to public school?''

''No, we've been sending him to a private school that specializes in hyperactive children,'' Mr. Castellano said, ''but to tell you the truth, I don't see that it's made that much of a difference.'' And then to the boy, the father yelled, ''Sit still, for Christ's sake!'' But Jeremy continued to kick the table.

''Oh, come on, Roger, he's much better than he was last year at this time,'' Mrs. Castellano said. ''Last summer, there would have been no way we could have kept him in this room for this long.'' No longer able to stand the noise of Jeremy's kicking and concentrate on the conversation at the same time, I tried to figure out a way to get and keep the boy's attention. Figuring Jeremy might be interested in my beeper, I unclipped old number 147 from my belt and handed the silver box to him. He took it eagerly, halting his torture of the table, and tried to figure out what to do with the thing. Mrs. Castellano broke the silence that followed: ''You know, I've been thinking; if my baby got sick because of a bad batch of formula, there must have been other babies who got it too. Did anybody else get sick?''

Miriam was saying, ''The company's had about a dozen reports of problems like Christina's,'' when Jeremy figured out how to trigger the beeper's test mechanism. The box made its high-pitched, irritating squawking noise while the nutritionist continued: "They're recalling every ounce of formula that came from that vat."

"There's talk that the Food and Drug Administration may force the company to take the product off the market completely," I added. Now Jeremy stood up, obviously disturbed by the sound the beeper was making, and started walking around the table, finally stopping in front of the window.

"Get away from that window!" Mr. Castellano shouted. Turning to look, I realized too late what was happening. In one fluid motion, Jeremy raised his right arm and, as I looked on in astonishment, lofted that beeper with its irritating noise right out the open window of the conference room. His parents, Miriam Doyle, and I rushed over and looked down. There, five flights below, in the middle of Harrison Avenue, lay the remains of my beeper.

Taking the steps two and three at a time, I made it down to the lobby in what must have been record time. Running out into the street, I retrieved my poor beeper: its top was smashed, the clip had broken off, and it was making a strange, terminal-sounding rumbling noise. Back in the hospital's lobby, I called the page operator and asked her to beep me. But it was hopeless: the box made no sound other than that sick rumble. Beeper number 147 had met its match: it never had a chance against Jeremy Castellano and his poor impulse control.

After returning to the conference room and finishing the discussion with Mr. and Mrs. Castellano, who were effusively apologetic, I nervously wandered over to the communications office. During our orientation session only a month before, a representative from the office had told us interns that we were each responsible for our own units, as she'd called them, and that if we were to lose or to damage the mechanism we could be charged up to $250. As I approached the office to report the incident, I fully expected the wrath of God to come down on me. But when I told the story to the supervisor, she laughed and said not to worry about it. "We have to expect these things to happen every once in a while,'' she said as she handed over my new issue, beeper number 226.

It had been early in my internship when I met Jeremy Castellano, and I'd still felt a great deal of responsibility for the care of my beeper. But as the year passed I came to learn that the little silver box clipped to my belt was my mortal enemy, rousing me anytime I had a chance to get some sleep, summoning me on a dead run from the bathroom when nature called, pulling me back into the hospital when I had the opportunity to escape. And when that realization hit me, when I understood the power that little box held over my life, not only did I come to see the beauty of the act Jeremy Castellano had performed that morning, I myself craved the chance to do it. Tossing it out the window was the thing I most wanted to do to my beeper; unfortunately for me, my impulse control had always been much better than Jeremy's.

The story I told satisfied the director of the communications office sufficiently to earn her initials on my Master Internship Release Form. More important, it allowed me to surrender my beeper permanently. With its loss, my life once again belonged to me. The lack of a beeper confirmed that I was no longer an intern; I had earned my freedom.

The pediatric department was sponsoring a party for us and our replacements. It was a festive affair: set up in the hospital's cafeteria, there was plenty of food and a good deal of alcohol, and nearly the entire house staff and faculty had turned up. I felt ambivalent about attending: on the one hand, the hospital was about the last place on earth I wanted to be, but on the other, I was one of the party's guests of honor. I decided at last to come, and I did try to have a good time, but I just couldn't bring myself to enjoy it. After only about fifteen minutes, I'd had more than enough.

I said goodbye to my fellow interns: I knew I'd probably never see most of them again, and quite frankly, this fact didn't upset me very much. We had been through a lot together, most of it unspeakably horrible, and I didn't have very many good memories. There were a few colleagues to whom I was truly sorry to say goodbye, but I knew I'd wind up staying in touch with them anyway.

And so, at a little after four o'clock, I walked out through the entrance of the Boston Medical Center for the very last time. Once free of the doors, I immediately headed for this bar, located just two blocks away from the hospital; happily, I found the place nearly deserted at this relatively early hour.

As I sipped at my beer alone in the dim light, I thought about the year that had just come to a close. I had come into my internship full of hope: that the experience would turn me into a real doctor; that I'd perfect all the necessary skills, learn all the vital information, gain all the practical experience; that after the sweat and tears and hard work I put in, I would come out able to call myself a physician. But as I sat in that bar, staring down at my beer, I knew I had failed.

I had gone in with hope, but I'd come away with memories: memories of nights spent without sleep; memories of wild, poorly run cardiac arrests that ended in death; memories of babies and children withering and dying as I looked on helplessly, unable to do anything to interrupt or alter the forces of nature, unable to do much of anything that made any difference at all; memories of residents and fellows and attendings who cared only about themselves, who didn't give a damn about what was happening to me, or to my fellow interns, or sometimes even to their patients; memories of the old me, the preinternship Bob Marion who had wanted to be a doctor because it might make a difference in people's lives, the Bob Marion who had been eager to read and learn about the conditions that afflicted his patients, the Bob Marion who had cared. And outside of approximately thirty sets of scrub suits, stolen from the surgical locker room on nights I'd been on call, these memories were all I'd have to take back to New York with me.

What had gone wrong? Why had it turned out this way?

As my third beer arrived I thought about it. Too many nights on call, too many hours spent in the hospital, those were the biggest problems; sleep deprivation and chronic exhaustion go a long way toward making people stop caring. There was no excuse for making interns work so many hours, no excuse except hospital finances; the system was dangerous to patients and destructive to doctors. Too little humanism, that was the next problem; in this internship, even if I had picked up a little medical knowledge and had come to feel comfortable drawing blood and starting IVs and performing spinal taps, I'd completely forgotten what compassion was all about.

I was getting tired; the excitement I had felt was wearing off, and the effects of the previous night on call were surfacing. I finished the beer and paid the bartender. Then I walked off toward the bus stop to catch the bus that would take me back to Watertown, where Beth and I would finish packing and get ready for the moving van that was scheduled to arrive in less than forty-eight hours.

PART III

Residency

16

Starting Over in the Bronx

First half of junior residency,
July–December 1979

At a little after nine o'clock on the morning of Friday,
June 29, 1979, two large moving men appeared at the
door of our apartment in Watertown. By noon, with a
little assistance from Beth and me, they had loaded all
our belongings onto their van and driven off. The next
morning, nearly two hundred miles to the south, the
moving men reappeared at the door of our new two-
bedroom apartment in one of the buildings owned by the
Schweitzer School of Medicine which sat on the campus
of Jonas Bronck Hospital. After twelve long months in
Boston, Beth and I had returned to New York.

For Beth, coming back to the Bronx was a welcome
relief. After developing her ulcer in the middle of October the year before, she had taken a leave of absence
from graduate school to spend the rest of my internship
year living in Watertown, finding little to occupy her
time. Through the previous spring she had grown increasingly restless, longing to get back to her work. Returning to New York meant that she would be able to
pick up her research and move toward finishing the lab
work required before she could begin writing her dissertation. During the first week of July, after the boxes were
unpacked, the furniture arranged, and we'd at least made

a start at settling in, Beth fished her white lab coat out of one of the wardrobe boxes, retrieved her notebooks, and returned to the laboratory at Columbia in which she'd spent the previous three years. By the start of August she had gotten her life back into a regular routine.

To me, the move back to the Bronx represented a major change. Residency is a marked improvement over internship in two important ways. First, the resident's on-call schedule is much more reasonable. Through all twelve months of my internship I had worked an every-third-night-on-call routine, a life-style that went something like this: on Monday morning I would go to work, staying in the hospital, constantly responsible for the well-being of my patients, until late Tuesday afternoon, when, after all my scut work was completed, I'd sign out to the intern who was scheduled to be on call that night; after signing out I'd rush home, able to do virtually nothing other than go directly to sleep; early on Wednesday morning I would report to work, staying in the hospital until the evening, when I'd sign out to the third intern on the team, the person scheduled to be on call that night; I'd spend Wednesday night relaxing, but then, come Thursday morning, I would report for work and, once again, would not be able to leave the hospital until thirty-six hours had passed. The schedule, which officially had me working between 100 and 120 hours a week, left me with little or no time for such basics as adequate sleep, let alone anything even resembling a social life.

Since I would be a second-year officer at Jonas Bronck Hospital, however, this routine would change. Residents in our program were scheduled to work every fourth night rather than every third, and that simple decrease in call made a radical difference in my life-style. Suddenly, from out of the constant, relentless grind that had characterized my internship, there was more free time; I was able to get more sleep, and to become reacquainted with my family and friends, many of whom, after having lost touch with me the previous summer, had assumed that I was angry at them, had developed a serious illness, or had simply vanished, without a trace, off the face of the earth; as a resident, I was even able to pursue some of my nonmedical interests—important parts of my life, such as reading and writing, that had been completely neglected during the previous year.

Second, in addition to the easing of the schedule, the start of residency creates a considerable change in duties. I was no longer required to spend my time doing the boring scut work that had filled the many hours of my internship. Scut work was in the job description of the intern, and, thank God, I was no longer an intern.

But becoming a resident didn't mean that my troubles were all behind me; with the start of that year came new, far more troubling responsibilities—tasks, it was true, for which less time-consuming mechanical work was needed, but which required a great deal more anxiety-provoking decision making. On the inpatient services, it is the job of the resident to supervise and guide the intern. As a resident, therefore, it was my responsibility to gather information about a patient's illness, to make a decision about the diagnosis, to provide a plan of management to correct the underlying problem, and to make sure the intern carried out the plan effectively. Early in the year, I discovered that the pressure to make those decisions as rapidly and accurately as possible accounted for why so many physicians developed prematurely gray hair.

In July I was scheduled, during my nights on call, to cover one of the pediatric wards at Jonas Bronck Hospital. Early in the evening of the fifth night of that month, the intern who was on call and I admitted an eight-year-old boy who had been brought to the emergency room by his mother because of lethargy that had gradually grown worse over the past few days. The mother had told the doctor who'd seen the child in the emergency room that, in addition to his lethargy, the boy had been drinking large quantities of fluids and urinating much more frequently than he ever had before, and although he had had a tremendous appetite and would eat everything in sight, he'd been losing weight. Recognizing the classic symptoms of diabetes, the ER doctor had obtained a sample of urine from the boy; the finding of sugar in the specimen had confirmed the diagnosis.

Testing of blood samples sent off once an intravenous line had been started showed that the boy's condition was serious. His blood sugar level was markedly elevated, and the tests showed that a buildup of acid had occurred in the boy's blood, a condition known as diabetic ketoacidosis, or DKA. The physicians in the ER then decided to admit the boy to our ward for treatment and careful monitoring.

"No problem," I thought to myself after I got the call from the emergency room informing me of this admission. "DKA's a cinch!" After all, during the three months of internship I had spent on the general pediatric ward at the Boston Medical Center, I'd cared for at least a half-dozen patients with diabetes who had come into the hospital with ketoacidosis. From that experience, I figured that I understood perfectly well exactly what needed to be done: while monitoring the blood, we would give this boy large quantities of intravenous fluids along with small amounts of insulin, the substance, missing or defective in diabetics, that allows sugar in the blood to enter the cells of the body, where it does its work; then, when the sugar level had fallen into the normal range, we would stop the infusion of insulin and add a little sugar to the IV solution. It all seemed very simple; but, of course, when I had been called on to do these things in the past, I was an intern, and I'd been told exactly what to do, as well as when and how to do it, by someone more senior than me. Now it was up to me to decide what had to be done and to supervise the intern as he went about doing it.

So, just to confirm that I'd gotten the treatment plan correct, while the intern went down to the emergency room to pick up the new admission I ran to the library to do some reading. Reviewing DKA in a textbook of endocrinology, I suddenly realized that the principles of management which had seemed so clear and straightforward when I had been an intern were, in reality, far more muddled and complicated now that I was a resident; the simple cookbook approach to diabetes I'd learned the year before was actually fraught with pitfalls. My review of the literature informed me that I needed to worry about a large number of very serious complications: if we corrected the blood sugar too rapidly, we might plunge the child into a condition known as diabetic shock; if we gave him too much IV fluid or ran the fluid in too rapidly, we could cause cerebral edema, or swelling of the brain, a potentially lethal disorder; and if we weren't careful we could cause disturbances in the boy's serum potassium level, which might result in life-threatening abnormalities in the rhythm of his heart. By the time I finished my reading, my anxiety level had risen dramatically; the feeling of confidence I had had on learning of this new patient's admission had disappeared, replaced by a queasiness in my gut.

I spent the entire night perched at the bedside of that eight-year-old boy. I watched the kid like a hawk; I told the intern what to do and when to do it, but I monitored the situation constantly. The next morning, after a night during which no serious complications had arisen, the boy's blood work revealed that he was much better: his serum potassium level was normal, his glucose was down in a much more acceptable range, and the IV fluids had successfully flushed the ketoacids out of his blood. The patient's condition was improved, the intern had managed to get three hours of sleep, but I was completely unnerved. It was clear that being a resident wasn't going to be as easy and painless as I had thought it would be.

But aside from the difficulties I had with the transition to increased patient responsibilities which accompanied the start of my junior residency year, nearly everything else about my life improved. Contributing to this improvement was the attitude of the people who ran the residency program at Jonas Bronck Hospital. From the day I first reported to work I was made to feel comfortable, and to know that there was somebody who was looking out for my well-being. I never felt that I'd been cast off on my own, forced to fend for myself against the many grim aspects of the house officer's life. On mornings after difficult nights on call, never once did I have to explain to an attending why some task that had been signed out the night before had not been completed; never once was I, or any of my colleagues, subjected to the kind of embarrassing, disrespectful put-downs in the name of discipline which had been so commonplace at the Boston Medical Center. The atmosphere of caring in the Jonas Bronck residency program helped make the hospital an enjoyable place to work.

But life as a resident in the Bronx was far from easy. The hours were still long, and I still spent most of my time chronically overtired. And there were some problems inherent in our community that at times made working at Jonas Bronck Hospital difficult. One of these factors was the complex social problems in the lives of many of our patients. The people who came to us for medical care were generally poor, and their poverty affected every aspect of their lives, including their health. Many of the parents of children who were brought to our clinics had simply given up, deciding it was easier to sit on the stoops of burned-out apartment buildings, drinking and collecting public assistance, than it was to go out every day and fight what amounted to a never-ending battle. Even for those who tried to escape the cycle of poverty, the social evils that characterized existence in the borough could prove overwhelming, as I learned one morning in the pediatric clinic.

17

One Morning in Pool

Middle of junior residency year,
January 1980

As I walked to work that morning, the ice and snow crunched under the soles of my shoes. The sky, gray and frozen, seemed to confirm the prediction of more snow on the way I'd heard on the radio before leaving for work: another major storm was expected to begin sometime during the early afternoon, and before ending twelve or so hours later, between six and eight new inches would be dumped on the Bronx. Huddled in my down parka, attempting to think warm thoughts, I imagined myself lying peacefully on a sunny beach in some island paradise. But as I approached the ambulance entrance to the emergency room of Jonas Bronck Hospital, my imagination failed to comfort me. It was January, the dead of winter, and my next vacation was still three long months away.

Entering the hospital, I caught a glimpse of the waiting area for the pediatric emergency room. The place was packed: at least twenty families were scattered around the room, families composed of exhausted-looking mothers, an occasional father, and one or two, or sometimes three or four children. The adults, who undoubtedly had been up most of the night, were lying on the hard plastic chairs, trying desperately to find a comfortable position in order to get a few minutes' sleep. Their children, both those who were sick and in need of medical care and those who were healthy but had been forced to come along because there hadn't been anybody available to watch them, tried to fend for themselves. I estimated the length of time most of them would have to wait before being seen by one of the residents who staffed the ER. "Five hours at the very least," I thought, passing through the door that led from the waiting area into the emergency room. But the backup wasn't my problem, at least not till afternoon. I wasn't scheduled to begin working in the ER until one o'clock, around the time the snow was scheduled to start falling, and I probably wouldn't be done until twelve hours later, well after the storm had blown out to sea.

Entering the emergency room, I found Phyllis Chambers, the senior resident working as night float, darting around the asthma booth, where four frightened, short-of-breath kids sat wheezing. Despite the fact that they were all wearing oxygen masks and receiving medication by mist, I could see that each child was still in significant distress. I approached the room and addressed Phyllis. "How are you doing?"

She stopped and, looking frazzled, stared at me. "I hate this place!" she said, collapsing onto the desk chair in the examining room next to the asthma booth and burying her head in her hands.

"What happened?" I asked, plopping myself down onto the chair beside the desk.

"I've got to get out of here!" she replied. "This is the first time I've even sat down since two o'clock."

"It's been like this all night?"

"No, things were fine until the paramedics brought in these two kids who'd been burned," she said. "They were sisters, two and four years old. The younger one was DOA; there wasn't anything we could do to get her back. But the four-year-old was still alive when they got here. She was in shock and she had burns over seventy percent of her body. A couple of the guys from the adult

ER and I worked on her for over an hour, but she was too far gone. We finally declared her at around three-thirty. By then, there were twenty-five patients waiting to be seen. I've been trying to catch up ever since, but I don't seem to be getting anywhere.''

I took a deep breath. ''How did they get burned?''

''Their bed caught on fire. The heat in their apartment had been turned off, and their mother had been using this old space heater to keep the house warm. It was so cold last night, she put the thing right up next to her bed and put the two kids in there with her. The heater must have shorted out or something. The firemen found them all huddled up together. The mother was declared in the adult ER.''

''Where's the early bird?'' I then asked.

''That's another thing,'' Phyllis replied. ''Okay, so I'd had a bad night, but when six o'clock rolled around, I figured at least I'd be able to go home and get some sleep. But then, just before six, Charley Simmons called; he's supposed to be the early bird today. He told me he had laryngitis and wouldn't be coming in. So what could I do? I couldn't argue with him for being sick. So I've been stuck here ever since.'' And then, as if I'd forgotten, she said, ''I really hate this place.''

''Well, the day crew should be here any minute,'' I said, but Phyllis just shook her head. I wanted to say something more helpful, something that would offer Phyllis some comfort, but I couldn't think of anything. Instead I got up out of my chair, walked into the nurses' lounge, and got her a fresh cup of coffee. ''Hang in there, it'll just be a little while longer,'' I said, placing the cup on the desk in front of her. And then I moved toward the exit and headed for the pediatric clinic.

The Pediatric Primary Care Center, the official name of the well-child clinic, had been the backbone of the pediatric residency program at Jonas Bronck Hospital since the program was founded in the fifties. The clinic, which was located in the basement of the hospital, served two major purposes: it provided quality medical care to the children of the Bronx at a fraction of the cost charged by private physicians, and it gave us interns and residents the opportunity to follow a group of patients we could consider our own while still in training.

The system employed by the clinic was simple: mothers of babies born in Jonas Bronck's delivery rooms were, on their infants' discharge from the nursery, offered clinic appointments. These new babies constantly feeding into the system were assigned to interns who, over the course of their first year of training, would establish a roster of patients. With the help of the attending physicians who were always available for consultation, the interns would give their little patients the immunizations mandated by the state's Department of Health; they'd offer mothers advice about their children's sleeping and feeding habits and about their development; the interns and residents were available when the kids became sick, watching, over the course of three years of hospital training, as the infants grew into children.

Occasionally the parents of children who hadn't been born at Jonas Bronck would make appointments to have their kids seen in the clinic. These children entered the system through a special clinic called "pool." Each morning and afternoon a different intern or resident would be assigned to the new patient pool to see these children who hadn't previously been followed in the clinic.

Because I had spent my internship in Boston and had returned to the Bronx only six months before, I hadn't accumulated a year's worth of newborns, and my roster of patients was much smaller than those of my coresidents. Thus during my rotations in the outpatient department, whenever I had a morning or afternoon free, I was almost automatically assigned to the pool. That cold January morning was no exception; once again, I'd drawn the job of pool resident.

Before entering the clinic area that morning, I stopped at the clerk's office to check the schedule. To my relief, instead of the full complement of five or six patients which was usually scheduled, that morning's pool list had only three names on it, members of a single family including two girls, eight and eleven years old, and their brother of fourteen. I quickly did some calculations: it took me about forty minutes to do a complete history and physical examination on an uncomplicated new patient; therefore, barring any difficulties, it would take me no more than two hours to finish my assigned work. That meant that after clinic, I'd have about two hours to try to sneak a nap before my marathon session in the emergency room was scheduled to begin. So without delay, I got down to work. Grabbing the charts that had been placed in my appointment box, I called the family's name over the loudspeaker and, when the family presented themselves in the corridor in front of the nurses' station, I silently led them down the hall toward one of the examining rooms.

The children were accompanied by their mother, a Mrs. Ayala. She was a short, heavyset, sad-eyed Puerto Rican woman whom I guessed to be about forty-five years old. During the first few minutes, Mrs. Ayala told me her story. She explained that she and her children were alone in New York, that her husband, no longer able to tolerate the poverty or the freezing cold of the Northeast, had abandoned them four years before, fleeing back to the warmth and relative security of Aricebo. Mrs. Ayala had a large family: parents, six brothers and sisters, and a multitude of nieces and nephews, but these relatives, too, were all back in Puerto Rico. She herself had considered returning to her homeland many times but had ultimately decided not to leave because, in spite of everything, she believed her children had a better chance of making good lives for themselves in New York than they would ever have back in Puerto Rico. So she'd remained in the cold city and tried as best she could to make a life for her family, working as a seamstress in a dress factory in the Garment District of Manhattan during the day, taking in laundry at night, and somehow keeping food on the table and clothes on all their backs.

When I asked her why she had decided to bring the children to the clinic that morning, Mrs. Ayala explained: "They have not seen a doctor in more than two years. I used to take them to a private man on Fordham Road. He gave them their shots and medicine when they were sick. But I have no money for him anymore. I decided they needed a checkup. So we came here."

I nodded, then asked, "Is there anything special that you're worried about with any of them?"

"No," Mrs. Ayala replied quietly, looking away.

So I began. Through trial and error I'd learned that, when examining multiple members of the same family, it usually worked best to start with the youngest. In this case that was Rosa, the eight-year-old, who was clearly the beauty of the family. With big brown eyes and long brown hair, she had a smile warm enough to melt snow. Thankfully, I realized almost immediately that Rosa was fine: after taking her complete history and doing a full physical examination, I declared her to be in excellent health, requiring only routine health care maintenance. And so, with only minimal protest from the girl, I placed a PPD, a test for tuberculosis, on her left arm and wrote a nurses' order for a routine complete blood count and urinalysis to be done. On finishing, I looked at my watch. It was nine-forty; so far, I was right on schedule.

Brenda, the eleven-year-old, came next. A sixth-grader, Brenda took after her mother; she was at least fifteen pounds overweight and much plainer than her sister, and she didn't smile at all; in fact, Brenda seemed to be completely empty of joy. I got her up on the examining table and began to take the history from her mother: "Has Brenda been in good health?"

Mrs. Ayala shrugged her shoulders. "She has been very sleepy lately, and she has too many bellyaches."

"Recurrent abdominal pain," I thought, writing these facts down in the girl's chart. She was just the right type for this problem, a disorder that most often is psychosomatic in origin: unhappy, overweight, and just beginning puberty, a triad of features I'd been taught occurred over and over again in girls who complained of frequent bellyaches. Dealing with these kinds of problems was frustrating; no matter how hard one worked at curing them, they never seemed to go away. As I gloomily finished taking the history from Mrs. Ayala, a history that did nothing to make me suspect there was anything more to Brenda's complaint, I began to plan in my mind the workup I'd have to perform and the long speech I'd have to deliver following the workup. "Oh, well," I thought to myself as I started the physical exam, "so much for my easy morning."

But while performing the exam, I realized that Brenda's problem wasn't as simple as recurrent abdominal pain. With her blouse off, the girl was, I saw, not simply overweight; her abdomen was definitely protuberant, though her arms and legs were as thin as her sister's. I felt a sinking feeling in the pit of my stomach as, with the girl lying flat on the examining table, I palpated the top of her uterus five centimeters above her belly button.

Involuntarily, I made a noise that must have sounded something like a groan. The findings on Brenda's examination shocked me, and I was pretty sure her mother would be just as shocked by the news. I didn't know exactly what to say to this woman, exactly how to put it; the sledding gets kind of rough when you're dealing with an eleven-year-old who's at least twenty-five weeks pregnant.

The examination completed, I asked Brenda to get dressed, then excused myself. I needed to regain my composure before continuing on. Walking out into the hall, I got a drink of water from the fountain, then paced up and down the long corridor of the clinic a few times, taking deep breaths along the way. I considered seeking help from one of the attending physicians, asking for advice about how to handle this situation. But I decided not to—I was a big boy now, and I had to work this problem out on my own. After reaching my decision and thinking through exactly what I was going to say, I returned to the examining room.

Brenda, now dressed, had glumly taken a seat next to her younger sister. "Mrs. Ayala, would you mind if we sent the children out to the waiting room for a few minutes?" I asked. "We need to talk." The woman had no objections, and the children were dispatched out into the clinic's waiting area.

"Uh . . . has Brenda started to get her period yet?" I asked tentatively.

"She got her first one six months ago," the woman answered blankly. "None since."

"Has she . . . does she have a boyfriend?"

"No," the mother replied quietly. And then there was silence for what seemed like an eternity.

I took a deep breath. "Mrs. Ayala, Brenda's about six months pregnant."

The woman made a hissing sound. But considering what I'd just told her, she didn't seem very surprised. "I know she is pregnant," the mother finally said after a long and uncomfortable silence. "I have tried to pretend it wasn't so, I have prayed it would go away, but I am not stupid, Doctor. I have seen what has happened to my daughter. I have seen her clothes get tight. I have watched her breasts get full. I know when a woman is with child."

"Why did you wait so long to come here?" I asked.

She shrugged her shoulders, and tears began to fill her eyes. "All my life I have worked," she said softly when she was again able to speak. "I have worked hard, and I have tried to do what is best for my children. I see what is happening in the streets, all the drugs and the stealing. I have told my children, I have told them all to stay away from the bad things, but what can I do? I have to work all day, I cannot stay home and watch them all the time. My girls, they are good, they listen to what I am saying, but my son, he thinks he does not have to listen to his mother; he goes out every day, and he gets mixed up with a bad crowd, with hoodlums, and then he gets into trouble. So I beat him, I hit him with a belt, and I tell him I will kill him if he gets into trouble again. And finally, he listens to me, he starts coming home every day right after school. And then, this . . .'' Unable to continue, tears now rolling down her cheeks, Mrs. Ayala finished her sentence by gesturing toward the ceiling.

I hesitated, trying to understand. ''You mean your son. . . ?''

She could say no words.

I was silent for a few seconds. ''It may be too late to do anything, to get an abortion,'' I finally began. ''It's not legal after twenty-four weeks, and it seems like Brenda may already be past that, but under the circumstances—''

''No!'' Mrs. Ayala interrupted. ''She cannot have an abortion. My religion says that abortion is murder, a mortal sin. No, Brenda will have this baby, and I will bring it up as my own child.''

''But her brother . . . it's dangerous. There's a good chance that the baby will be born with serious birth defects.''

''What my son did was a sin, but it is done, and there is no way to stop it now. This is a sin I can do something about.''

''Mrs. Ayala, maybe if you were to speak to your priest—''

''No, Doctor, nobody will change my mind. We have to do what we have to do.''

Mrs. Ayala and I spent the next two hours in the examining room. I tried again and again to convince her of the danger to Brenda, both medically and psychologically; I told her of the problems that could occur in the unborn baby, and what effect this pregnancy might have on little Rosa. We discussed the legal implications: her son had sexually abused Brenda, a criminal offense, and I told Mrs. Ayala that it was my duty to report the incident to the Bureau of Child Welfare, the New York State agency that handled cases of child abuse. But the mother pleaded with me not to turn the boy in; she asked that I leave the disciplinary action to her. Realizing that the boy, this whole family, would need prolonged, intensive professional help, I made a deal with the woman: I told her that I would hold off reporting the case to the authorities if she would promise to talk with the clinic psychiatrist that morning and make it her business to bring her son and the other members of the family back for as many visits as the psychiatrist thought they needed. Reluctantly, the woman nodded her head.

We both agreed that it was time to end, that we'd all had enough for one morning. I gave Mrs. Ayala my beeper number in case she needed me, or just wanted to talk, but I had the feeling she wouldn't call it. I handed her a referral slip to the hospital's prenatal clinic so that Brenda could register for the obstetric care she would need. And finally, I walked the whole family over to the psychiatrist's office. Saying goodbye at his door, I worried that I'd never see any of them again.

I had to talk. After dropping the Ayalas off, I suddenly felt the need to seek out someone, anyone, and tell this story, to get what had happened off my chest. Walking into the consultation room, I found the place deserted except for Jack Stevens, my old friend from medical school. Jack, who was also then a junior resident, was sitting on one of the consultation room chairs, gazing out the window, apparently lost in thought.

"It's snowing," I said, looking out the window and noticing the infrequent flakes.

"Yeah," Jack replied dreamily, after some hesitation. "It started a couple of minutes ago."

"What are you doing in here all by yourself?" I asked.

"Just thinking." He sighed.

"Boy, I just had a really bad case," I said, launching into a full account of the Ayala family's story.

Continuing to gaze out the window at the falling snow, Jack didn't interrupt or make any sign that he even heard what I was saying. When I had finished spinning out the entire tale, he began one of his own: "I just saw these

two kids I've been following since last year," he began.
"A one-and-a-half-year-old boy I picked up at the start
of internship and his five-year-old sister. They came for
their regular visit today. Their grandmother brought
them, because their mother died two weeks ago. She got
into an argument with the kids' father, and he took out
a gun and shot her in the head. Now she's dead, he's on
Riker's Island, and they're living with their grandparents."

"Jesus!"

"And that's not even the worst of it," Jack went on,
still gazing out the window. "These poor kids saw the
whole thing. They watched their father blow their mother's brains out. Can you believe that?"

Unfortunately, I could believe it, just as I could believe
the story of Brenda Ayala, and the one Phyllis Chambers
had told me in the emergency room earlier that morning
about the family that had been burned to death. These
incidents had become all too familiar: kids suffering because of what life in the Bronx, in all inner-city ghettos,
had done to them. Our patients lived in apartments with
no heat or hot water or electricity; they ate the paint and
plaster chips that fell from the ancient walls and ceilings
and got lead poisoning; their only pets were the mice
and rats who ran unrestricted through the kitchens and
bathrooms, eating whatever they could find, and when no
food was available, gnawing on the fingers and toes of
the little ones who hadn't yet learned how to fight them
off; they watched as junkies shot up and died before their
eyes, on the stoops and in the alleyways; they sweltered
in the summer and froze in the winter. And we, the interns and residents of the pediatric department at Jonas
Bronck Hospital, we who served as their doctors, were
supposed to try to keep them healthy in spite of all this.
At times, our job was as frustrating and unrewarding as
that of Sisyphus.

In a few minutes, Jack rose and left the room. I continued to look out the window, watching the snow, now
falling heavily and more consistently, begin to accumu-

late on the ground, covering the dirty brown stuff that had lain there for days as if a fresh white blanket had been unfurled, a blanket that hid below it all the dirt and grime and ugliness of this horrible city.

I gazed out the window for a long time, in total silence. And then, returning to the empty examining room, I collected my coat and backpack. With a sigh, I headed back up to the emergency room, where the pile of charts of patients waiting to be seen had grown significantly taller.

One night in May of that year I was working as the cross-covering resident in the neonatal intensive care unit at Jonas Bronck Hospital. Besides keeping an eye on the critically ill patients in the Intensive Care Unit from Hell, the intern and resident on call were required to perform admission physicals on all the healthy babies who were born since the evening began. So, around midnight, the intern assigned to the unit and I walked down to the well-baby nursery, where we began to make our way through the half-dozen or so new admissions.

Having examined my third patient, I went out to the maternity ward to talk with the baby's mother and to reassure her that everything seemed to be all right with her newborn baby girl. Standing over the mother's hospital bed, I immediately recognized the features of the sleeping face, the face of a child rather than of a woman. Sleeping in that bed on the postpartum ward was Brenda Ayala, and the infant, this Female Child Ayala whom I'd just finished examining, was her daughter. The child, who'd been born around nine o'clock that evening, weighing a little over six pounds, seemed to be perfect in every way.

During the course of the intervening four months, I'd spoken with Brenda's mother three times. The conversations had all been phone calls, and each call had been instituted by me so that I could check that the woman was holding up her end of the bargain. I could tell that Mrs. Ayala didn't welcome my calls; although she was always civil, she was also very curt, never telling me any more than the barest of essentials: yes, they had been keeping their appointments with the clinic psychiatrist; yes, her son had seemed to be making progress; no, there had been no complications in Brenda's pregnancy. But that had been it.

I stood over Brenda's bed for a few seconds, watching her sleeping face. I thought about waking her, seeing how she was feeling, finding out if there was anything I could do for her. But because she looked so peaceful, I decided against it. Letting her sleep, I walked back to the well-baby nursery to start on the next examination.

The remainder of my junior residency year passed without incident, and in July of 1980 I became a senior resident, at long last entering my final year of medical training.

There was very little difference, I soon found, between being a junior and a senior resident. The call schedule was every fourth night for both years, and although the senior resident was given some additional responsibilities (for instance, the senior resident took charge and ran the emergency room; the junior resident was responsible only for seeing patients), the job description remained pretty much the same.

I can, however, point to one significant difference between my junior and senior residency years. As a senior resident, I spent two consecutive months supervising the interns assigned to the pediatric service at University Hospital, a rotation from which junior residents were exempt. Working at University Hospital, a private facility run by the Albert Schweitzer School of Medicine and located in the middle of the Schweitzer campus, was a lonely experience; except for the three interns who were assigned to the ward with me, the rest of the house staff was back at Jonas Bronck, and the four of us thus had little contact with our fellow interns and residents.

Other than the loneliness, working at University Hospital wasn't bad. The patients were interesting, free meals

late September. Prior to entering University Hospital, Kathleen had been a normal nine-year-old girl who only two weeks before had begun fourth grade. She had been in excellent health until that afternoon, when after returning from school, she'd been playing with a group of her friends on the sidewalk in front of the apartment building in which she and her mother lived in the south section of New Rochelle. The girls had been playing a game with a rubber ball. At some point the ball had careened away from them, out into the street, and Kathleen had run to retrieve it.

From what we'd come to understand, after speaking with the police, Kathleen's mother, and some of the girl's friends, it had all happened amazingly fast. She hadn't stopped to look before running into the street; she apparently never saw the car, a large gray Mercedes, that had been heading north on Pelham Road, traveling at thirty miles an hour, the legal speed limit on this heavily traveled street that connected the Pelham Bay area of the Bronx with the Westchester suburbs. The driver of the car, Dr. William Westergreen, a senior orthopedic surgeon at University Hospital, was on his way home from work. Later he told the police that he hadn't seen the girl until it was too late to either slow down or stop. The impact with the heavy car, which had struck her squarely, launched Kathleen ten feet straight into the air. Returning to earth, she landed on her head; by the time Dr. Westergreen had pulled his car over to the curb, gotten out onto the street, and joined the pack of children who had rushed to the girl's side, Kathleen had already lapsed into a deep coma.

The scene became a mass of chaos. Some of the children, mainly Kathleen's closer friends, began crying wildly when they saw what had happened; others crowded around the girl, staring at her, unable to take their eyes off her apparently lifeless body. Luckily, a group of adults had been standing nearby; one of them immediately went into the apartment building to call for an ambulance while another, a friend of the family's, went up to get Mrs.

Warrington, Kathleen's mother. After learning of the accident, Mrs. Warrington came running; she rushed into the street, to her daughter's side, where, faced with the stark reality of the situation, she began to scream. Mrs. Warrington tried to move Kathleen out of the gutter, but Dr. Westergreen, who was huddled over the girl's body, blocked the mother's advance. "Don't move her," he told her. "She should not be moved. Don't even touch her."

This speech caused Mrs. Warrington to tip over the edge. Shrieking "Get away from my baby, get away from my baby," she began hitting Dr. Westergreen, pummeling his shoulders and back with her fists. She continued her attack for nearly a minute, until some of her friends dragged Mrs. Warrington out of the street and back into the sidewalk.

Horrified by what had happened, by what he and his car had done, Dr. Westergreen had tried to keep a level head. On reaching Kathleen, he had removed his suit jacket and covered the girl with it; he'd made sure that she was breathing on her own (at that point, she had been) and that her heart was beating at an adequate rate (it was); and then he'd briefly examined her. He understood when he saw the head wound, the deep gash on the right side of the girl's skull through which blood was flowing at a slow but steady rate, how devastating such an injury could be. Having set the broken bones of uncounted patients who had suffered similar trauma, the orthopedic surgeon knew that the large laceration, the apparent point of contact between Kathleen's body and the surface of Pelham Road, was probably hiding a deeper, more profound and horrible injury. Beneath this gash, Dr. Westergreen knew, pressing on the area with his handkerchief in a feeble attempt to stop the flow of blood, lay the sensitive, unprotected brain of this nine-year-old girl, a brain that had probably been severely, perhaps irreparably damaged by the impact.

Unable to do anything else, the orthopedist knelt beside the girl, monitoring her vital signs, waiting for the

ambulance to arrive. During the entire period Westergreen did not say another word to Mrs. Warrington, who,
crying inconsolably, stood off to the side, supported by
one of her neighbors, helplessly looking on at the scene
in the street.

After about fifteen minutes an ambulance finally arrived. The two paramedics worked fast: they first placed
heavy sandbags on either side of the girl's neck in order
to stabilize her cervical spine; then, very carefully, they
loaded her onto a gurney; and less than ten minutes after
they'd arrived, with Kathleen's mother, still crying, on
board and with Dr. Westergreen following close behind
in his Mercedes, they drove off to New Rochelle Hospital.

There, in the emergency room, Kathleen was evaluated by the physician on call, who, like Dr. Westergreen,
had instantly recognized the severity of the girl's head
injury. According to the reports we received, the ER doctor had sprung into action. First, to ensure that she could
breathe, he carefully intubated Kathleen, passing a plastic breathing tube down into her trachea, making sure
not to move her neck, which was still sandbagged, even
an inch while doing so. Next the ER physician started a
large-bored intravenous line in the girl's left arm; then,
using a pair of sharp, heavy-duty surgical scissors, he
and the nurses cut away Kathleen's polo shirt and jeans
in order to allow them to examine the girl's entire body
without obstruction. Finding only superficial cuts and
bruises on her legs and trunk, with no additional signs
of serious internal injuries, the ER doctor was satisfied
that only the head wound required immediate attention.
He then took the girl down to the radiology suite, staying
with her while a series of X rays of her head and neck
were taken. On his way to the radiology suite, the ER
doctor was approached by William Westergreen. "What
do you think?" the orthopedic surgeon asked.

"I think this is a very sick little girl," the ER doctor
said coldly.

"Is there anything I can do?"

"Pray, if you think praying does any good," was the response.

"I have a friend who's a pediatric neurosurgeon—" Westergreen began.

"Well, get him the hell over here right away," the ER doctor replied as he disappeared through a door, pushing the gurney in front of him.

So, while Mrs. Warrington, who had been led into the family room by one of the hospital social workers, kept crying, Dr. Westergreen called the office number of his old friend, Dr. Jeffrey Sheldon, the pediatric neurosurgeon at University Hospital. He and Dr. Sheldon had known each other for years, and they'd scrubbed together in the operating room on a number of spinal injury cases. "Jeff will know what to do," Westergreen thought to himself as he dialed the number.

And sure enough, Jeffrey Sheldon knew exactly what to do. When the call from Dr. Westgreen came in, Dr. Sheldon was just finishing his regular Friday afternoon office hours. "Jeff, I'm in some deep shit here," the orthopedist said, and Sheldon, never having heard his friend us a four-letter word, recognizing the panic in his friend's voice, replied, "Stay right where you are, Bill. Don't move an inch. I'll be there in a few minutes." After hanging up, the neurosurgeon quickly went to his car and headed north for the emergency room entrance of New Rochelle Hospital.

Dr. Sheldon reached the ER just as Kathleen Warrington was being wheeled back from the radiology suite by a nurse and the ER doctor. After greeting his friend, who, having taken Sheldon's advice literally, was still seated in the same position in the nurses' station, the neurosurgeon performed a quick but complete physical exam on the girl. Dr. Sheldon's chart note reflected the fact that he had first noted that Kathleen was deeply comatose, responding to nothing, not even sharp pain; he'd also noticed that the joints of her arms were flexed, positioned close to her chest, that her hands made tight fists, and that her legs were rigid and extended. Recog-

nizing that this pattern was consistent with decorticate
posturing, a sign of severe, diffuse dysfunction of the
cerebral cortex, Dr. Sheldon came to the same conclusion that the ER doctor had reached after his own examination: that, below the neck, Kathleen Warrington
was probably perfectly fine, but above the neck she had
been transformed into a major neurological disaster, a
case requiring expert neurosurgical attention.

After examining the girl Dr. Sheldon hurried to the
radiology suite, where, with the ER doctor and the radiologist on call, he reviewed the X rays that had just
been taken. Methodically searching among the black and
gray shadows, lit by the bright light of an X-ray viewbox,
Sheldon noted that, although Kathleen's cervical spine
appeared normal, her skull showed a large fracture underlying the site of her laceration. Worse still, a piece of
bone from the fracture site had indented, like a crushed
Ping-Pong ball, as a result of the impact with the street;
the X ray clearly showed that this fragment of bone was
directly pressing on a portion of the girl's brain. "A depressed fracture," the neurosurgeon said on seeing this
formation, pointing out the shadow to the ER doctor and
the radiologist. "We have to get this kid into an operating room right away."

That's when Sheldon really went to work. Cutting
through as much of the red tape as he could, he took care
of all the arrangements: he called the operating room
supervisor at University Hospital and told her to prepare
a room for emergency surgery within an hour; he phoned
the hospital's intensive care unit and reserved a post-op
bed; he called the admitting office and told them of this
new emergency admission; and finally, he ordered the
emergency room clerk to get an ambulance to the front
door of New Rochelle Hospital, stat. When all the arrangements were completed, he went into the family
room, where Mrs. Warrington was sitting, no longer crying but obviously very agitated and nervous, and introduced himself to the woman.

"Is Kathy going to be all right?" the mother asked.

"Your daughter is very sick," Sheldon replied. "She's suffered a very serious head injury."

"It's all my fault," the mother interrupted, her voice louder, the tears again spilling over and falling down her cheeks. "I should never have let her go out into the street by herself like that. She's only a baby, and the streets are so busy now—"

"She needs a very delicate operation," Dr. Sheldon continued, ignoring the mother's comments. The neurosurgeon explained what needed to be done: he told the mother about the depressed skull fracture, how if the fragments of bone weren't delicately lifted off the brain and the covering of the brain repaired, permanent damage would almost certainly result.

Jeffrey Sheldon had no trouble convincing Mrs. Warrington of the necessity of the operation; he got her to sign a consent form, allowing him to perform the necessary procedure at University Hospital. "Will Kathy be okay after the surgery?" the mother asked after setting down the pen.

"Only time will tell," Sheldon responded philosophically.

In less than an hour, Kathleen Warrington was lying on a table in an operating room at University Hospital. While her mother, intermittently crying softly to herself, and Dr. Westergreen, chain-smoking, paced nervously around the OR waiting room, not uttering a word to each other, Jeffrey Sheldon performed the delicate two-hour-long neurosurgical procedure. Opening the skin around the girl's large wound, he irrigated the area with a solution of sterile saline into which a broad-spectrum antibiotic had been mixed until the entire region appeared free of dirt and debris. Then, carefully, he lifted the dented-in piece of bone which impinged on the girl's right cerebral hemisphere, exposing a small patch of her brain. This was Dr. Sheldon's chance to see the damage the injury had caused to the girl's brain. He looked closely, using an operating microscope to see the fine structures more clearly. But the microscope wasn't really necessary; the Surgeon watched helplessly as, right before his eyes, Kathleen Warrington's cerebral cortex swelled up like a dry sponge dropped in a pale of water; in seconds, that small segment of brain expanded to occupy all the space just vacated by the newly removed chunk of bone.

The swelling that occurred in Kathleen's brain, though very serious, was not unexpected. Cerebral edema, the medical term for brain swelling, is a common consequence of serious head injury. It can cause the pressure within the skull to increase dramatically, a phenomenon that can literally squeeze the life out of the brain.

The skull, a hard, bony case designed to protect the brain, can't itself expand or contract. In addition to the brain, the skull contains two other essential components: blood, which brings nourishment to the cerebrum; and cerebrospinal fluid, which cushions the brain against injury. When the volume of one of these three components increases, the volume of the others must somehow diminish. In cerebral edema, increased volume of the brain caused by swelling, leads to increased intracranial pressure, which essentially stops the flow of blood. No blood going to the brain means that the organ will get no oxygen or glucose, the essential nutrients needed for cerebral function, inevitably causing the brain to wither and die. So, although Dr. Sheldon had successfully repaired her depressed skull fracture, Kathleen Warrington, following her neurosurgery, was only beginning the struggle that would determine whether she ultimately lived or died.

After noting the presence of cerebral edema, Jeffrey Sheldon promptly took action. He ordered the anesthesiologist, who had been closely monitoring Kathleen's vital signs and respirations during the surgery, to increase the girl's breathing rate; he then ordered that she be given a very large dose of phenobarbital, a common anticonvulsant. Finally, the neurosurgeon drilled a small hole in the left side of the girl's skull and implanted a catheter, a plastic tube that would be used to constantly monitor the pressure within her head.

After finishing his work, Dr. Sheldon personally brought Kathleen up to the hospital's intensive care unit, where we, the pediatric house staff, had our first chance to see the girl. I happened to be on call that night, and I distinctly remember my reactions on laying eyes on her: first I groaned; then I had the genuine desire to kill myself.

My reactions were based on two facts that were very clear even on first glance. There was the realization of how sick Kathleen Warrington was, and what her illness would mean administratively in the running of the pediatric service. Still in decorticate posture, the top of her head covered with a gauze turban that hid her surgical site, there was, projecting from the left side of the turban like one of the antennas that rose from the head of Ray Walston in his role of Uncle Martin in the sixties television series "My Favorite Martin," the intracranial catheter Jeffrey Sheldon had placed into position in the OR only minutes before. Although I knew that this catheter, which was hooked up by wires to one of the most complex monitors I had ever seen, would provide us with essential information about the girl's well-being, the machine would also make slaves of my interns and me. One of us would always have to be present at the girl's bedside in the ICU, constantly monitoring the pressure readings, waiting for the numbers to edge up into the danger zone, when immediate action would need to be taken. By manipulating the settings on the ventilator to which Kathleen had been attached, by giving her massive doses of phenobarbital, by cooling her body temperature down to 95°, and when the pressure rose acutely, by squirting a few grams of the diuretic mannitol into her intravenous line, we could keep her intracranial pressure within the normal range. But the price we would pay was that a member of the team would have to be assigned to Kathleen alone, leaving the rest of us with lots of extra work to do.

The second reason for my reaction was my knowledge of what it was like to work closely with Jeffrey Sheldon. I had heard rumors about the man since returning to the Bronx from Boston the year before. At unpredictable moments, the rumors had it, for reasons only he could explain, Dr. Sheldon was known to devise all sorts of cruel torture for the persons with whom he worked. In the operating room, it was said, on more than one occasion he had thrown scalpels and other sharp surgical instruments at the house officers who were assisting him. He had also once attempted to fire a secretary who had worked for him for more than five years simply because she was pregnant and had had the nerve to ask for a three-month maternity leave—a guaranteed benefit. But I myself hadn't had the opportunity to deal directly with Dr. Sheldon until the Sunday before Kathleen's admission, during the first week of my two-month rotation at University Hospital.

I had been sitting in the nurses' station, minding my own business, passing the time by doing the Sunday *New York Times* crossword puzzle, when my beeper went off. It was an outside call, so I picked up the phone and, dialing the number specified by the page operator, said hello.

"Is this the pediatric senior resident?" the male voice on the other end asked, and after I confirmed that it was, he continued: "This is Dr. Sheldon. Do you have any problem with beds?"

"No," I replied without giving it a second thought. "We've got plenty of room."

"Great," Dr. Sheldon's voice replied. "There's a baby over at Bronx Episcopal Hospital I need to transfer in. His name's Rodriguez and he's three months old. He's a preemie who had an intracranial hemorrhage when he was a week old, and now he's got bad hydrocephalus. I'm planning to take him to the operating room tomorrow morning to put in a ventriculoperitoneal shunt. You got all that?"

"Yeah," I answered, jotting the information down at the bottom of one of my sign-out sheets. The neurosurgeon had described an infant born prematurely who had suffered a hemorrhage into his brain, the equivalent of a stroke. The hemorrhage, an all-too-common complication of prematurity, led to an obstruction in the path taken by cerobrospinal fluid through the infant's head and into his spinal cord, resulting in hydrocephalus, a buildup of fluid within the cavities of the brain. The only way to treat hydrocephalus is to place one end of a piece of plastic tubing, called a shunt, into the fluid-filled brain cavity and the other end into another body cavity, usually the abdomen, allowing the fluid to drain from the head into the relatively low-pressure environment of the peritoneal cavity. "I'll tell the nurses he's coming," I continued. "When can we expect him to get here?"

"The doctors in the Episcopal nursery assured me they'd handle all the details," Sheldon answered. "Knowing those guys, it'll take at least two hours for them to figure out the phone number of the damned ambulance company. I wouldn't plan on the kid getting there much before seven or eight tonight. It shouldn't be any big deal, but I'd like you to do a favor for me."

Because of the stories I'd heard about Dr. Sheldon, my first impulse was to tell him to shove it. But I successfully fought off the urge, replying instead, "Sure. What is it?"

"I wonder if you'd mind calling the admitting office and letting the people down there know that the baby's on his way," the neurosurgeon. "Just tell them to admit the kid to my service. Okay?"

"No problem," I responded. I assured him that I would handle it, then hung up. As I dialed the number of the admitting office, I thought for sure I could handle it. Hell, by September of my senior residency year, after nearly two and a half years of being a house officer, I was certain that I could handle anything. By then I could perform all the technical tasks required of a pediatrician, from starting an intravenous line in the tiniest baby to doing an all-out cardiopulmonary resuscitation on anything that had a heart and lungs; and I could handle all the administrative headaches that were part of the job, everything from conning an abusive and hostile lab technician to run a critical blood test in the middle of the night to getting dinner for the interns and me delivered from the Chinese restaurant down the street which offered no delivery service. I thought I could do anything, but I was wrong. On that day I was to be brought to my knees; on that afternoon, I nearly met my administrative match.

When the weekend clerk in the admitting office answered the phone, I told her that I needed to admit a patient to Jeffrey Sheldon's neurosurgical service.

"Okay," the clerk said. "What's the patient's name?"

"Rodriguez," I replied, and without prompting, I answered the other questions I knew she was going to ask: "He's three months old, his diagnosis is hydrocephalus, and he's coming as a direct transfer from the neonatal intensive care unit at Bronx Episcopal Hospital. I don't know anything else about him, either his address or his phone number, but I'll give you a call with that information as soon as he gets here." And then I fell quiet, sure that I had supplied all the information that could possibly be needed. But then the admitting clerk asked a question I wasn't prepared to answer: "What's the patient's first name?"

"His first name?" I repeated. "I don't know."

"We need a first name in order to admit him," the clerk replied.

I thought for a second. "Okay," I said. "I'll call Bronx Episcopal and find out."

I looked up the hospital's number in the telephone directory. After a few minutes of frustration with the hospital switchboard, I found myself speaking with the clerk in the NICU. "You want to know about Baby Rodriguez?" she asked when I said I was calling from University Hospital. "We've just managed to reach an ambulance company." Verifying Jeffrey Sheldon's prediction, she added, "It took us a long time to find their phone number, but they told me they'd get here within an hour or so.''

"Right," I replied. "Look, our admitting office wants to know what the baby's first name is. It's just a formality, but—"

"Rodriguez's first name?" the clerk interrupted. "Hold on, Doctor." She put the phone down; in the background I heard some muffled voices, then some laughter. Finally the clerk came back on and said, "I'm sorry, Doctor. Everybody here says that Baby Rodriguez doesn't have a first name. His mother's a junkie, and after he was born she never came around to see him. She never gave him a name. As far as we know, he's just Male Child Rodriguez."

"If the mother's not around, how did Dr. Sheldon get permission to do the surgery?" I asked.

"Oh, that's easy," the nurse replied. "The baby's a BCW case." He'd been referred to New York State's Bureau of Child Welfare, the agency in charge of investigating cases of child abuse and neglect. "The doctors here got permission for the operation through them."

I thought about this for a few seconds. "Okay, thanks." I hung up, then redialed the number of the admitting office. "That patient I called you about a little while ago doesn't have a first name," I told the clerk after I had again identified myself. "He's just known as Male Child Rodriguez."

"We can't admit a three-month-old child without a first name," the clerk responded. "Isn't there some way you can contact the mother?" I then proceeded to repeat for her the story I had been told by the Bronx Episcopal NICU clerk.

"Well, I don't see that there's anything I can do," she said after I had dramatically unfolded the whole episode. "We're not permitted to admit a patient electively without a full first and last name."

"But this is an emergency—" I attempted.

"Is Dr. Sheldon planning to take the child to the operating room today?" she interrupted.

"No," I replied glumly, knowing she had me. "He's not scheduled until tomorrow morning."

"Well then, he qualifies as an elective. And as I said, for all elective admissions we need a full name. You'll simply have to contact a family member."

I began to feel a headache coming on. I had spent about fifteen minutes trying to work out a solution to this puzzle, but there appeared to be no way out. After a few more minutes of thought, I decided to give Dr. Sheldon a call.

He answered on the third ring. "Dr. Sheldon," I began, "this is Bob Marion, the senior resident at University Hospital. I'm having a little trouble getting that Baby Rodriguez admitted."

"What kind of trouble?" the attending asked, obviously not happy that his Sunday had been interrupted.

"Well, the admitting office requires a first name on any nonemergency patient," I explained.

"Yeah?"

"Well, Rodriguez doesn't have a first name. I called Bronx Episcopal, and the clerk there told me his mother never—"

"I don't think I understand—" he interrupted.

"Yeah, I don't understand the rule either," I interrupted back. "It seems dumb to me but—"

"No, I don't care about the stupid rule. I was going to say that I don't think I understand why you're bothering me with this. I asked you to take care of admitting this patient, and I thought you told me you'd do it."

"Yeah, I did, but—"

"Dr. Marion, I don't think I'm asking you to do anything beyond your capabilities here, no matter how limited those capabilities might be. I'm not asking you to do the surgery or anything like that. It doesn't seem too much to ask to get a single patient admitted to the hospital, Doctor."

"Well, I didn't think it would be too much to ask either, until I started dealing with—"

"Look, I'm going to be in that operating room at eight

o'clock tomorrow morning, and I expect that baby to be in there with me. I don't care what you have to do; all I know is, it better get done!'' He hung up the phone.

By then, my head was pounding. ''Why do these things happen when I'm on call?'' I asked myself. ''Other people are on, they get hit with admissions, they work their asses off, they get the job done, and then they go home. When I'm on call I wind up sitting here doing nothing all day except fighting with a jerk neurosurgeon, and torturing myself with the idiotic admitting office. Who the hell gives a shit what this kid's first name is?''

That rhetorical questoin changed the complexion of the day. At that moment I realized that nobody did give a shit what Male Child Rodriguez's first name was; nobody, that is, except me. His mother apparently didn't care, the clerk and nurses at the Bronx Episcopal NICU didn't care, the neurosurgeon didn't care; the admitting clerk cared only that the baby had a first name, not what that name was. And so I decided to give Male Child Rodriguez a first name.

Before calling the admitting office I considered a good many options: the theme of the crossword puzzle I had been working on before this mess started was Greek mythology, so I first tried some of those names. But Prometheus Rodriguez just didn't have the proper ring to it. Next I thought about some of the common Hispanic first names, such as José, or Eduardo, or Jorge. Somehow, though, they all sounded—well—too common. It occurred to me next to name the kid after myself: ''Robert Rodriguez,'' I thought; ''not bad.'' But the longer I considered it, the less I liked the idea of forever linking myself with this unfortunate child.

And then, like an inspiration, the answer came to me: why not name the child after the man who was going to save his life? I knew it was the right thing to do the moment it entered my mind. Without delay, I proudly dialed the number of the admitting office and, when the clerk picked up the phone, said, ''Good news: I managed to reach Male Child Rodriguez's aunt. His name is Jeffrey. Jeffrey S. Rodriguez.''

From then on, the admission process proceeded like a well-oiled machine. Within two hours, Jeffrey Sheldon Rodriguez had reached the pediatric floor. He had his blood drawn and his IV started, and the next morning his hydrocephalus was corrected by the most important man in his life, the neurosurgeon who not only put in his shunt but also gave him his name.

Besides learning that afternoon that I wasn't as invincible as I had thought, I also came to realize that, when everything in life is considered, a name simply isn't all that important; it really was true that a rose by any other name would smell as sweet. But just try convincing an admitting clerk of that in the middle of a Sunday afternoon and you'll spend your life arguing with jerks like Jeffrey Sheldon, who'll want you to explain to them why they have to operate on their patients in the hospital parking lot.

For the first three weeks following the accident, Kathleen Warrington remained in a deep coma, lying in the decorticate posture she'd settled into soon after she hit the ground, unresponsive to all external stimuli. She wasn't aware of her mother, who, having taken a leave from her job, stayed by the girl's side almost constantly, talking to her, touching her skin, believing that these things would force the girl to react in some way, to show signs of life. She wasn't aware of the many cards she'd received from her classmates, friends, and relatives, mail her mother brought from home and taped to every existing inch of wall space surrounding the girl's ICU bed. She never saw Dr. Westergreen, who, guiltily, came to check on her three or four times a day. During his visits the orthopedic surgeon spoke to no one, not a word to Kathleen or her mother, or to the nurses and doctors caring for the child; he would simply enter the unit, stand by the nurses' station, and check the vital sign sheets kept by the nursing staff; after a few minutes had passed, he'd walk out of the unit. Sometimes there was a tear in his eye as he left.

And Kathleen wasn't aware of us, the pediatric house staff, the doctors in charge of her day-to-day management, as we went about our work. She didn't cry or withdraw when one of us drew blood from her arm; she didn't react when we flashed lights into her eyes or poked her in the legs with pins in an attempt to test her mental status and the deepness of her coma. To us doctors, who had never seen her in any other state, Kathleen was nothing more than a brain stem preparation; she was a human being who had lost, possibly forever, the part of her brain that made her human in the first place. To us, the girl was as inanimate as a mannequin.

But however inanimate, during the first two weeks of her stay in the ICU Kathleen required much more management than any department store dummy. During those weeks the pressure inside her head, monitored constantly on the sophisticated internal catheter system Dr. Sheldon had installed at the time of surgery, remained persistently elevated. Despite doing everything we knew of to keep it in the normal range, her intracranial pressure repeatedly skyrocketed to dangerously high levels. These flare-ups of hypertension required rapid action: when they occurred, we would immediately squirt large doses of mannitol into the girl's intravenous line. Usually Kathleen responded readily to this treatment; within minutes of administering the drug, the readings on the pressure monitor would sink back toward normal. But since these episodic blips on the monitor screen came unpredictably and without warning, six, seven, even eight times a day, it had become necessary for one of us essentially to move into the ICU to maintain a constant watch over her at all times.

The job had fallen to Tom Johnson. As the intern on call the night Kathleen was first admitted, Tom had become her primary physician. Although initially he had dreaded the time he was forced to spend baby-sitting this apparently hopelessly ill girl and her monitor, by the end of the second week he had come, if not exactly to enjoy it, then at least to tolerate the task. Through the many hours of boredom he began to make friends with Mrs. Warrington, a nice but lonely woman who had, with the loss of both of her parents, a messy divorce from her husband, and most recently this terrible accident that had befallen her daughter, endured a great deal of sorrow over the past three years. Tom also enjoyed watching the activities of the ICU, the life-and-death dramas that were played out every day in the unit. He even looked forward to the frequent weird visits of Dr. Westergreen.

What Tom and the rest of us didn't look forward to were the daily visits of Jeffrey Sheldon and his neurosurgery team. The case had evidently taken on a special meaning for Dr. Sheldon. It wasn't just a simple case of head trauma; it was a case of head trauma in which one of his old friends had also been traumatized. The neurosurgeon always seemed angry when he came to see Kathleen, frustrated that she wasn't responding to therapy. As the days passed and the possibility that Kathleen might never awaken from her deep, sound sleep grew, Dr. Sheldon became angrier and even more irritated; roaming the ICU during rounds, he would search for a scapegoat, a victim on which he could blame the girl's poor response, on whom he could take out his growing rage.

But it didn't seem that he would ever seize on Tom Johnson as that scapegoat. Because he'd become so attached to Mrs. Warrington, Tom had taken meticulous care of Kathleen. He made sure that every blood test was drawn and checked at precisely the right time; he ensured that every electrolyte imbalance and alteration in the girl's oxygen and carbon dioxide levels were promptly and accurately corrected. On work rounds each morning, as we spent nearly an hour reviewing what had happened to Kathleen the day before, Tom amazed me with his ability; I wasn't sure whether Kathleen Warrington had even a chance of surviving this severe head injury, but I knew that if she did make it, it would largely be owing to the excellent care Tom Johnson had given her.

Although the first two weeks were difficult and there were times when we were sure that Kathleen would not survive, gradually, over the course of the third week, the girl's condition began to stabilize, her intracranial pressure at last coming under control. When, near the end of the third week, three days passed since she'd last needed a dose of mannitol to reduce her pressure, we began to withdraw some of the extraordinary measures we'd been taking. We first tapered the amount of phenobarbital Kathleen was receiving. With the decreasing level of the drug in her blood, she became "lighter"; although still in a coma, for the first time she moved her arms and legs spontaneously, finally moving out of decorticate posture on the twentieth day after the accident. The acute phase of her illness was over, and so, three weeks to the day after the accident had occurred, Dr. Sheldon took the girl back to the operating room and carefully removed the intracranial pressure catheter.

Things began to look up for Kathleen. But then, during her fourth week of hospitalization, her progress inexplicably stopped. She had plateaued, remaining comatose and continuing to rely on the mechanical ventilator to provide her with oxygen. She never once responded to her mother's attempts to communicate with her, which caused Mrs. Warrington, whose spirits had briefly risen around the time the catheter was removed, to fall into a deep, dark depression.

Kathleen remained like that, vegetative, through the entire fifth and sixth weeks of her hospitalization. Sometime during that period, Dr. Westergreen stopped visiting; never having said a word to Kathleen's mother, or to any of us, the orthopedic surgeon must have decided one day that he'd had enough torture. We didn't find him hanging around the ICU again.

And sometime during those fifth and sixth weeks, Jeffrey Sheldon became even more frustrated and angry. He would yell at the neurosurgery residents who worked with him, especially Dan Santos, the chief resident, who, through some bizarre thinking, Dr. Sheldon had begun to blame directly for Kathleen's lack of progress. Sheldon's words, shouted at the chief resident so that everyone in the ICU could hear, insulted Santos's surgical skills, his family, his ethnic background, even his manhood. Somehow Santos, with an enormous amount of self-restraint, took Sheldon's abuse in stride; not once did he fight back or argue.

Meanwhile, sometime during those two weeks, each member of our team came to accept the fact that Kathleen had settled into a chronic vegetative state from which she'd probably never emerge. Even Tom Johnson, who continued to do everything he could for the girl, understood that his hard work would most likely be in vain. I too believed that Kathleen's condition wouldn't change, that she would remain trapped in the ICU, her heart beating and oxygen being pumped into her lungs by machine, until arrangements could be made to move her to a chronic care facility. That's what I thought, but that morning, during our work rounds on the pediatric ward, something had apparently changed. I rushed toward the ICU, knowing that something terrible must have happened to Kathleen Warrington.

We came running into the unit at top speed. Being the first to enter, I threw open the double doors and headed off to the left toward Kathleen's bed as Tom Johnson and the others followed close behind. All the while I was reviewing in my mind the routine normally followed after a patient has had a cardiac arrest.

By the time I made it to her bedside I was ready to begin resuscitating Kathleen. But when I pulled to a stop, I saw I had been wrong. Kathleen hadn't arrested; she was as stable as she'd been at any time during the previous month; the cardiac monitor showed that her heart was still pounding away in her chest, and the ventilator continued to force air into her lungs. No, her condition hadn't deteriorated, not in the slightest. Then why had we been called to this bedside, stat? That's when I noticed Jeffrey Sheldon.

He was standing just above the head of Kathleen's bed. In his eyes was anger; in his mouth was a Tootsie Roll lollipop (he'd been trying to give up cigarettes for some time, and he said that he needed to have something in his mouth). Sucking hard on his lollipop, he'd surrounded himself with a few neurosurgery residents. Although Sheldon was obviously furious, angrier than I had ever seen him before, it was difficult to take him seriously: that lollipop stick dangling from his mouth made it awfully hard for him to strike fear into our hearts.

Before beginning, the neurosurgeon waited until all six of us had assembled by Kathleen's bedside. "Who's in charge of this patient?" he finally yelled, pointing the index finger of his left hand toward Kathleen.

Without hesitation, both Tom and I raised our hands. "Do either of you have any idea what the results of this morning's blood gas were?" Sheldon asked, anger in his voice.

"Sure," Tom answered. "The pH was seven-point-forty-four, the pCO_2 was thirty-three, and the pO_2 was eighty-nine." I nodded when I heard these results; the two most important parameters, the pH, which measured the amount of acid and base in the blood, and the pCO_2, the amount of carbon dioxide, were both right where we wanted them; the quantity of oxygen suspended in the blood, the pO_2, was also within the acceptable range.

But these results did not elicit from Jeffrey Sheldon the same feelings of joy that they'd brought forth in me. "What was that pO_2 again?" he growled in Tom's direction. "Would you mind repeating that number?"

"Eighty-nine," Tom repeated, adding the following editorial comment: "Completely acceptable."

"Eighty-nine's completely acceptable, huh?" the neurosurgeon mocked. "Do you agree with that, Dr. Marion?"

I nodded. Sheldon's voice rose: "So the pediatric house

staff believes that a pO_2 of eighty-nine in a head trauma patient is completely acceptable! No wonder this patient hasn't regained consciousness yet. She's being cared for by a staff of idiots, of fucking morons, of shit-headed know-nothings!'' Turning toward one of the neurosurgery interns, Sheldon asked, ''Shapiro, can you tell us why a pO_2 of eighty-nine is not acceptable in a head trauma patient?''

''Studies have shown that the prognosis for patients with head trauma who have increased the intracranial pressure is markedly decreased if their pO_2 falls below ninety.'' The intern responded as if he'd been programmed—which he probably had.

''Correct,'' Sheldon said. The attending's face was now bright red. ''I thought everybody knew that. But apparently the fucking pediatricians, the people who are in charge of the medical management of this patient, don't even have a clue about it. You know what? I'm embarrassed. Do you know why I'm embarrassed?'' Without waiting for a response, he went on, his voice growing louder and louder: ''I'm embarrassed because in New York City, in New York State, in the Middle Atlantic states, in fact, along the entire eastern seaboard, I am considered the leading expert in pediatric head trauma. And to have a patient of mine treated so poorly, by shit-headed doctors who don't even understand the importance of maintaining the pO_2 above ninety, is a profound embarrassment to me!'' And with that, the neurosurgery attending stepped away from Kathleen's bedside and walked out of the ICU. In silence, the neurosurgery residents followed close behind.

Shocked by this outburst, and feeling bad for Tom, who had been singled out by the jerk Sheldon, I asked if he was okay. ''Sure; I'm fine,'' the intern replied. ''Why should I be upset?''

''Well, Sheldon just gave it to you pretty good,'' I answered.

''You think I'm going to become unglued because a

maniac who's sucking on a lollipop yells at me that the pO$_2$ is eighty-nine and not ninety? That guy's just nuts!''

Of course Tom was right. No matter how many studies the neurosurgeons could cite, the human body cannot recognize the difference between an oxygen level of eighty-nine and ninety. Kathleen Warrington was still in a coma because the injury she'd suffered had been so severe; her condition had nothing to do with the care she had received.

Leaving the ICU, our team walked slowly back to the pediatric ward to continue work rounds. Before departing, I asked Tom if he wanted to make any changes in Kathleen's ventilator settings to increase the amount of oxygen being provided. Flashing me an angry look, the intern didn't respond.

At four o'clock the next morning, Kathleen Warrington opened her eyes and asked the nurse who was checking her blood pressure for a drink of water. Since it was the middle of the night, the nurse wasn't sure if she'd actually heard Kathleen saying those words or if she'd just imagined them. She asked the patient to repeat her request. ''Could I please have some water?'' the girl clearly asked.

She had awakened. Just like that, with no provocation, without any special assistance from us, the neurosurgeons, or anyone else. In the middle of the night, after six weeks spent who knows where, Kathleen Warrington was back with the program.

The intern on call was awakened. After verifying that this seeming miracle had really occurred, she called Kathleen's mother in New Rochelle, waking the woman out of a deep sleep. Mrs. Warrington, who'd been waiting for this call, dreaming about it night after night, told the intern that she'd come as soon as she could get dressed. At a little after five o'clock that morning, Kathleen Warrington and her mother had a touching, tearful reunion in the ICU.

When he heard the news on arriving at the hospital

two hours later, Tom Johnson was ecstatic. Rushing into the ICU, he hugged both Mrs. Warrington and her daughter, squeezing both of them tight for minutes. During work rounds we made Kathleen's bedside our first stop, and for the first time the team met the little girl who'd seemed little more than a mechanical torture device during the previous six weeks. We all came to know that morning that there was a little girl in that ICU bed, one who had been terribly sick and was now better. As we left the unit, all of us, the interns, the medical students, and I, were beaming from ear to ear.

In the hall outside the unit, as we were heading back toward the pediatric ward, we ran into the neurosurgery team, led by Jeffrey Sheldon and Dan Santos, the chief resident. "Did you see Kathleen?" Dan asked with a broad smile on his face as we passed.

"Yeah," I replied, smiling back at the chief resident, trying hard to ignore the existence of his attending. "It's great, isn't it?"

"Absolutely," the chief resident said. "She isn't out of the woods yet; she still has a long way to go, but at least she's conscious. You guys deserve a lot of credit. You took terrific care of her. If it hadn't been for you, Tom, I don't think this ever would have happened."

Tom blushed, and he almost said, "Aw, shucks." But instead it was the voice of Jeffrey Sheldon we all heard. "Santos, how can you compliment that schmuck for doing a good job when, less than twenty-four hours ago, I yelled at him for doing such a shitty one?" Sheldon had a slight sneer on his face, and I wasn't sure if he was joking or not.

"You yelled at him yesterday?" Dan Santos asked the attending physician, the smile suddenly leaving his face.

"Yeah, I yelled at him for letting the pO_2 drop below ninety. Where the hell were you?"

Dan thought for a moment. "I must have been in the OR during that emergency case. Gee, I'm sorry—"

Sheldon cut the chief resident off. "I don't want to hear about your being sorry. Next time I yell at someone,

I want everybody there. I don't want to have to explain who I yelled at, and why I yelled at him the next day, do you understand?'' And with that, the neurosurgeons passed down the corridor, the team disappearing into the ICU.

I wasn't around when Kathleen Warrington stood for the first time, or when she took her first step. Her recovery took many months and, only ten days after she had regained consciousness, our team finished its two-month rotation and we all moved on to other hospitals. But I stayed in touch with the residents who worked at University Hospital in the months after my rotation had come to an end to keep up with the girl's progress. Just a little over four months after her nearly fatal accident on the streets of New Rochelle, Kathleen Warrington walked out the front door of University Hospital to return to her life as a normal suburban preadolescent.

The tongue-lashing Tom Johnson received in the ICU at University Hospital from Jeffrey Sheldon was, in many ways, similar to the one that Kevin Donahue, the head of hematology and oncology, had given me on the general pediatric floor at Boston Medical Center two years earlier. Both attacks had been launched because of complaints regarding patient care; both had occurred in front of a crowd of interested people; and just prior to both, the victim had been summoned to the site of the attack by beeper. But the results of the two attacks were very different: Tom Johnson simply shrugged off Jeffrey Sheldon's words, whereas Kevin Donahue's had wounded me deeply. The more I've thought about it, the more I've come to realize that the different reactions Tom and I had stemmed directly from the different characters of the two training programs.

In October of his internship, Tom Johnson had much more confidence in his abilities than I'd had at the same point in my internship. Through the preceding months, Tom had been built up by the people around him; he'd been praised by the directors of the program for the good job he'd done rather than constantly criticized for the tasks he was unable to perform. Thus when he was confronted by Jeffrey Sheldon in the ICU that morning, Tom understood that the problem existed only in the mind of the neurosurgeon, not in the quality of work that he had done.

During my own internship, through the actions of the faculty who ran the program, I had come to believe that blame for just about everything ultimately rested on the shoulders of me and my fellow interns. Naturally, when I was attacked by Kevin Donahue, I assumed that I was at fault. The more I thought about these two incidents, the happier I was with my decision to return to the Bronx for the last two years of my training.

As the rest of that senior residency year passed, my confidence climbed to astronomically high levels. By March I thought I knew everything there was to know about pediatrics. Of course, I was wrong.

19

Meningitis

**Approaching the end of senior residency,
March 1981**

After finishing my examination of the baby I sat back
down on the desk chair and began the speech I had already delivered to at least fifty sets of parents during the
course of that day: "It looks as if your son has a bad
case of the flu," I began wearily. "There seems to be a
lot of it going around. There's nothing we can do to make
it go away; it just has to run its course. This particular
strain of flu has been lasting about five or six days from
start to finish, and since your son has already been sick
for three days, it should only be another couple of days
before he's back to his old self. In the meantime, make
sure he gets plenty of fluids, and give him a dropperful
of infant Tylenol every four hours if his fever comes
back." Then, without waiting for a response from the
eleven-month-old boy's mother, I started writing my
findings on his ER sheet.

"That's it?" the woman asked after a pause. "I spend
three and a half hours out in that damned waiting room,
I expose my baby to all those other sick kids out there,
and all I get out of it is a lousy speech about giving him
plenty of fluids and Tylenol? I could have stayed home
and gotten that advice from watching TV commercials!"

"I'm sorry you had to wait three and a half hours to

be seen,'' I replied slowly, looking up from the chart, ''but as I said, a lot of kids came in today, and most of them seem to have the flu.'' The woman's attention was focused on forcing her son back into the bulky snowsuit he'd been wearing when they first arrived in the emergency room, but I could feel the rage directed toward me. ''I'd love to make your son's flu go away right now, I really would,'' I added, ''but there isn't anything I, or any other doctor, can do. I'm sorry.'' And with that, I looked back down at the ER sheet and continued writing.

''Shouldn't he be on an antibiotic or something?'' the woman asked, her voice rising. She'd gotten the baby's snow pants back on and was attempting to pull the heavy jacket over his shoulders. The child, obviously not thrilled about the idea of getting back into all those heavy winter clothes, was squirming around and howling irritably. In order to be heard over the racket, the mother was now shouting at me. ''The pediatrician I usually take him to puts him on an antibiotic whenever he gets like this,'' she pressed.

That's when I nearly snapped. I had been working without a single break since eight o'clock that morning, more than fourteen hours before; I'd been second-guessed, manipulated, and straight-out yelled at by a steady stream of angry, hostile parents who, like this woman, had found themselves having to wait hours and hours before their sick children could be seen; parents who, when their children's charts finally reached the top of the pile in the triage box and they had been seen by a doctor, were told that there were no magic bullets, no drugs or chemicals or other mysterious hocus-pocus that I, or any of the other residents on call that day, could prescribe or administer or incant which would immediately alleviate all the fevers, muscle aches, sore throats, and other symptoms. I had had it, and I could no longer sit back in an understanding and sympathetic way and just take it. So I lashed out: ''Well then, the pediatrician you usually take him to is doing the wrong thing,'' I exploded, standing up and staring into the woman's eyes.

"Antibiotics don't work for viral infections; they only work for bacteria. The flu is caused by a virus, and viruses just don't get better with antibiotics."

"Oh, so you think you know more than our pediatrician, huh?" the woman shouted back angrily. She lifted the baby, who, now completely re-dressed in his bulky winter clothing, resembled a screaming, squirming version of the Pillsbury Doughboy. "You're only a resident, right?" Without waiting for a response from me, she went on: "And you think you know more than a doctor who's been in private practice for over fifteen years? You don't know anything! But I know something; I know that I'm never, ever coming back to this hospital! I'd sooner let my baby die in the street than have to go through what we've gone through tonight again!" And with that she turned and, carrying the crying Doughboy in her arms, headed out toward the waiting area.

"Looks like another satisfied customer, Marion," said Cynthia, the head nurse. She had come running when first she heard the woman raise her voice and stayed around to make sure a fistfight wouldn't break out.

"I just don't understand these idiots," I exclaimed, shaking my head, my voice still raised in anger. "If this woman has a regular pediatrician she trusts and is happy with, why the hell is she dragging her poor sick kid out to the emergency room at Jonas Bronck Hospital on a freezing cold Saturday night?"

Cynthia replied without hesitation. "Because pediatricians in private practice don't see patients on Saturday nights. If your kid's sick and you try to call them for advice, you get hooked up to their answering service, where the operators have been instructed to tell you to take the kid to some emergency room for evaluation."

"Well, that's not right," I said, my voice starting to return to normal volume as I turned my attention back to the baby's chart and attempted to finish the paperwork. "If you're a family's doctor, you should be their doctor all the time, not just weekdays between nine and five."

"Face it, Bob," Cynthia said, "that's the way it is.

On Saturday nights, we're the only game in town. Gives you a feeling of power, doesn't it?''

"Power, nothing. It makes me crazy. These sixteen-hour days here during flu season are insane, just insane. I can't take too much more of this. Are there many more patients out there?''

"We're still about two and a half hours backed up. But trust me; everybody out there just has the flu. Hang in there, Bob. It's already after ten; the night float will be here in less than two hours.''

"Two hours,'' I sighed. And then I rose and walked to the nurses' station to pick up the next patient's chart.

It was the beginning of March and I was the senior resident in charge of the Jonas Bronck pediatric emergency room that day. Cynthia's reminder that the night float was due to arrive at midnight went a long way to settle me down. I knew I could survive working in the emergency room for a measly two more hours; hell, I could survive just about anything for two hours. So, my spirits at least temporarily buoyed, I completed the chart for the eleven-month-old, dropped his papers into the clerk's OUT box, and pulled a fresh chart from the top of the half-full waiting-to-be-seen box on the triage nurse's desk. "Jesus Christ, another flu," I muttered to myself as I hastily perused the nurse's note which had been scribbled at the top of the chart three hours before: DANIELLE THOMPSON, it read, NINE-MONTH-OLD WITH FEVER OF 104°, LETHARGY AND VOMITING SINCE THIS MORNING. Shaking my head at the thought of having to go through the routine with yet another parent, I called Danielle's name into the microphone and leaned against the triage desk, trying to keep my eyes from closing while I waited for mother and child to make their way to the emergency room.

It wasn't long until Ms. Thompson, a frazzled, tired-looking woman, appeared at the entrance to the emergency room. She was clutching her daughter, who was wrapped in a blanket and crying irritably, in her arms. The woman couldn't have been more than twenty years old. I signaled for her to follow me and walked to the examination booth I'd been using. Ms. Thompson took the seat across the desk from me. "The baby's sick," the woman said softly before I'd even had a chance to introduce myself. "I'm worried about her."

"She probably just has the flu," I replied matter-of-factly. "Everyone seems to have it today. She's had the fever since this morning?"

"Yes," the mother said, "and she's been very sleepy and cranky like this all day. She hasn't had much of an appetite; I've had to force her to eat, and she's vomited everything I've fed her anyway. She's just not acting like herself. You really think it's just the flu?"

"It sure sounds like it," I said, trying to sound reassuring. "Let me take a look at her." I directed the mother to undress the baby and place her on the examining table.

But when I saw Danielle lying naked on the table, I knew there was something terribly wrong with her. She lay there limply, her muscle tone very poor, while she shrieked in a high-pitched, pained voice, the kind of voice I'd heard before only in infants and children with serious neurological problems like hydrocephalus or meningitis, a sound so shrill and eerily frightening that it sent chills down my spine. The girl's temperature was so high that I could feel the heat rising from her as I stood by, looking down at her body. I got a queasy feeling in my stomach; this child had something far more serious than a simple case of the flu.

With only a moment's pause to catch my breath, I set about examining Danielle. I tried to bend her neck and found that it was as stiff as a board. When I put my hand behind her occiput, the back part of her skull, and lifted, the girl's shoulders raised up clear off the table. Propping her head up and cradling it in my left hand, I felt the anterior fontanelle, the soft spot of her head, with the fingers of my right hand; rather than being flat or sunken, as it should be in a child Danielle's age, it was bulging, and it pulsated in and out with each beat of her too rapidly contracting heart—sure signs of increased pressure within her skull.

That bulging, pulsating fontanelle clinched it for me. Danielle Thompson had meningitis, a life-threatening infection of the fluid and membranes that surround and protect the brain; I had no doubt about it. As the elements of the treatment plan that would have to be begun over the next three or four hours passed quickly through my tired mind, I realized that the night float coming at midnight couldn't offer me the relief I had longed for. Since I had started this case, there was no way I could sign it out; I was going to have to do the workup myself, including performing a spinal tap, drawing blood, and getting a sample of urine for culture. When the workup was completed, I would have to start an intravenous line and push large doses of antibiotics into the baby's bloodstream; then, after the antibiotics were run in and the child's condition had stabilized, I would need to examine a specimen of the spinal fluid under the microscope with eyes blurred from exhaustion, counting the hundreds or thousands of white blood cells I was sure would be present. But the workup and treatment were the easiest parts of my task. Sometime during the small hours of the morning it would also be my job to tell Ms. Thompson, to whom only minutes before I'd been so casually reassuring, that her daughter could die or, at the very best, with intensive care during the next few weeks, be left severely and permanently brain damaged.

"It is the flu, isn't it, Doctor?" the mother asked, the sound of her voice shattering my musings.

I hesitated. "It might be," I replied finally, now cradling the baby in my arms, "but I'm a little concerned it might be something else—"

"What else could it be?" the mother interrupted, a look of panic flashing into her eyes for the first time.

"I think the baby might have meningitis," I answered.

The mother's eyes now opened wide. "Meningitis," she repeated in a quiet voice. "My baby's got meningitis?"

"She might," I said. "She has some of the symptoms. We'll have to do some tests to find out for sure."

"What kind of tests?" the woman asked. I could see tears beginning to form in her eyes.

"Some blood tests and a spinal tap," I replied. "And the faster we do it, the better off Danielle will be. I think it would be best if you'd wait outside while I start to get ready—"

"Are you sure this is necessary, Doctor?" The woman was almost pleading with me.

"Yes, I'm sure." I led her out of the examining booth. "Just have a seat out in the waiting room. I promise I'll come and talk to you as soon as I'm finished doing the tests."

"She's going to be all right, isn't she?" the woman asked as she began moving toward the waiting area. The tears now ran freely down Ms. Thompson's cheeks.

"Sure, she'll be just fine," I said with as much conviction as I could muster as I signaled for Cynthia to come over. "Now just go have a seat and try to relax. I'll be out to talk to you in a few minutes."

I had lied to that woman; I was sure her daughter wasn't going to be just fine. I'd seen other children who looked like this, kids who came into the emergency room with high fevers and irritability and necks as stiff as this baby's was. The spinal taps on these children yielded fluid that was as white and thick as pus; under the microscope, these fluids revealed thousands of white blood cells and entire civilizations of bacteria. These kids were immediately admitted to the critical care unit, where they received massive intravenous doses of antibiotics for two full weeks to ensure that the infection was completely eradicated. But this intensive care nearly always came too late; the damage had already been done by the time the children first stepped through the doors of the hospital. I'd taken care of these children during my rotations in pediatric neurology and in developmental medicine. I'd tried to control their seizures with drugs and diets that almost always proved ineffective. I had attempted to

find school programs suitable for these severely neuro-
logically impaired children, had looked on as physical
therapists, trying to make their limbs functional again,
manipulated their stiff, frozen joints, and had realized
their howling was the only way some of them would ever
respond to external stimuli. I knew all this, but I hadn't
told Ms. Thompson about it. I had lied to her, reassured
her, told her that everything was going to be all right
because I couldn't tell her the truth—not just then, not
in the state of exhaustion I was in. So, as I plopped this
beautiful baby onto the examining table and got ready to
perform the spinal tap that I was sure would confirm the
diagnosis and seal her fate, I silently prayed that my impression was wrong, that Danielle really did only have a
bad case of the flu, that when I stuck my needle through
the skin of her back and popped it into her spinal canal
the fluid that would gently leak out would be crystal clear
and free of white blood cells and bacteria—that the baby
would go home with her mother and lead a normal,
healthy life, never having to learn about CT scans and
electroencephalograms, about anticonvulsant levels and
signs of toxicity, about special school programs and New
York City's Committee on the Handicapped. But I was
certain I was right.

Cynthia was silent while she helped me. She had
worked in the emergency room a long time and knew
exactly what was happening. She held the shrieking, irritable baby tightly as I drew a specimen of blood for the
complete blood count and cultures that were part of the
routine workup for meningitis. The infant didn't change
the pitch or the intensity of her crying when my needle
passed into her elbow. Then, while I was shooting specimens of blood into the appropriate tubes, the nurse positioned Danielle for the spinal tap: expertly she turned
the girl on her side, held her arms and legs tightly, and
flexed her back out toward me. While pulling on a fresh
pair of sterile gloves, I said, "Cindy, I'm getting too old
for this."

"That's why internship and residency training only lasts three years," the nurse answered.

After washing the baby's back with a sterile cleaning solution, I grabbed hold of the spinal needle. I held it firmly between the thumb and middle finger of my right hand while my left thumb felt around on the child's back for the exact location of the space between the fourth and fifth lumbar vertebrae. "Okay, hold tight," I said after I was sure that I'd located the spot, "and pray."

The nurse squeezed the child and closed her eyes. I eased the needle through the skin of the girl's back and slowly, slowly advanced it until I felt the familiar pop. I gently removed the needle's inner cannula, and fluid began to fill the hub of the needle. As the liquid dropped into the sterile tube I'd placed beneath the needle, both Cynthia and I breathed sighs of relief. The fluid was as clear as glass.

My training was drawing to a close. In January I had accepted a postresidency job as a fellow in human genetics, and I was eager to get on with the rest of my life. By May, I was counting the days until I would no longer have to spend every fourth night in the hospital; around the middle of June, I was down to counting the hours.

During that June, while working in the emergency room at Jonas Bronck Hospital, I came across an old acquaintance, a child named Albert Wilson. That meeting with Albert and his mother came as a surprise; after our last meeting, I never thought I'd see either of them again.

20

The Return of M/C Wilson

Last month of residency,
June 1981

When I called his name over the loudspeaker, the kid came barreling through the doors in a matter of seconds. He looked somewhere between four and five. While I waited for his mother to catch up with him, I glanced down at the ER sheet to see if I was right.

Close, I discovered, but no cigar. The kid, whose name was Albert Wilson, was barely three and a half, and obviously large for his age. He'd been brought to the emergency room that night, according to a note on the chart written by the triage nurse, because of a rash on the skin of his left arm which had been present for the past month or so. A one-month-old skin rash!

This kind of case used to drive the old me crazy. It could be the middle of the night, there could be a huge backlog of patients waiting to be seen, and a mother or father, for some inexplicable reason, would choose that time to bring a child who'd been complaining of a skin rash, stomachache, constipation, or some other chronic annoyance for at least a few weeks, sometimes even a couple of months, into the emergency room. In the past, whenever the triage box had dealt me one of these families I would call the patient and his parents into my examination room, sit them all down, and when I was sure they were comfortable, let the parents have it: "This is an emergency room, for Christ's sake, not a walk-in clinic!" I'd begin. "We're here to provide care for emergencies, not for little aches and pains that have been going on for months; you can make an appointment in the clinic for things like that. If your child had a real emergency, how would you like it if you had to sit around waiting while the doctors took care of other patients who had skin rashes?"

The parents, who by now would most likely be staring down at their shoes, wishing that their kid's chart had been picked out of the triage box by one of the more sane ER doctors, would inevitably choose not to reply to this question. After an awkward silence I would continue, browbeating them for a while longer until, having relieved myself of much of the aggression and aggravation that had built up during the course of the shift, I would shut up and set about taking care of the child's presenting problem. After my speech I would always treat the kid; after all, it wasn't the patient's fault his parents had little or no sense at all.

But that had been the old me. The change to the new me hadn't been caused by experience, or by the fact that I'd once uncovered some dreadful, life-threatening problem in a child who'd been brought in because of three months' worth of bellyaches. No, I was different simply because I was coming to the end of my residency. It was the middle of June, I had only nine days of work left, only two more nights on call in the emergency room, and I was feeling no pain. "They can't hurt me now," I had repeated to myself for the previous month or so, a kind of end-of-residency mantra that had helped me get through these last few days.

And so, when Albert Wilson's mother appeared behind her three-and-a-half-year-old son at the door of the emergency room, I welcomed her, led her to a seat in the examination room, and instead of treating her to one of my usual tongue-lashings, very sympathetically began to gather information about the little boy's rash. "When did you first notice it?" I asked.

"About six weeks ago," Ms. Wilson replied as she sat the boy down on her lap. There was something familiar about the woman, but that didn't surprise me; after months of working in the emergency room, clinics, and wards of Jonas Bronck Hospital, I felt as if I'd met the mother of nearly every child who lived in the Bronx at least once. "One day, there wasn't anything there. The next day, when I was giving him his bath, there it was."

"Has it been itching?"

"Not that I know of," the woman replied. The boy, who was very well behaved, continued to sit quietly on his mother's lap; so far he'd been a pleasure compared to most of the three-year-olds I'd dealt with that day. "He doesn't complain much about it. I probably wouldn't have brought him in at all, except it's been there for so long and it doesn't seem to be getting any better."

"I'd better take a look at it." I had the woman take off the boy's shirt. There, on his upper left arm, was a circular lesion about the size of a quarter; in the center, looking like a target, was a clear, scaly region, a patch surrounded by a peripheral ring of small raised vesicles. "Ringworm," I said. "It's nothing to be concerned about, but you were right to bring him in. Ringworm is caused by a fungal infection, and Albert needs medication to get rid of it. I'll give you a prescription for some lotion." While the mother was putting the boy's shirt back on, I wrote out the prescription.

"Rub this stuff on the spot three times a day," I instructed, handing over the prescription form. "It'll probably take a few weeks for it to go away completely, and it might actually look a little worse before it disappears entirely. But don't worry if it does; that's just part of the normal healing process. Okay?"

Without waiting for a response, I began to write out the history and physical on the boy's ER sheet. But I looked back up when the mother asked, "So, how do you like the way Albert turned out?"

"He looks fine," I said with a smile, not understanding what the woman meant.

"Yeah, he is fine. But that's not how you and all the other doctors said he was going to turn out when he was a baby," the woman responded.

"Did I take care of Albert when he was a baby?" I asked, a little puzzled.

"Yeah, you were one of them," she replied.

"I don't think so," I said quickly. "I was only a medical student when Albert was born. You might have me confused with one of the other doctors."

"No, it was definitely you," the woman insisted. "You used to talk to me a lot about him when he was in intensive care. None of the other doctors did that, especially after that heating thing broke and Albert got so sick."

Then I realized who Albert Wilson was.

During the last two weeks of my elective rotation as a fourth-year student in Jonas Bronck Hospital's Intensive Care Unit from Hell, Male Child Wilson had held the distinction of being the sickest patient in the place. He'd been a preemie, born twelve weeks before his mother's due date and weighing just a little over a pound and a half at the time of his birth. As a newborn, M/C Wilson suffered most of the usual complications of prematurity: he developed respiratory distress syndrome and required the use of a mechanical ventilator for weeks; the immaturity of his liver causing jaundice, had resulted in a buildup of the chemical bilirubin in his blood, and he had to be placed under special neon "bili" lights for days and days; and he had sepsis, a serious bacterial infection in his blood which was treated over a period of two weeks with high-dose, broad-spectrum intravenous antibiotics. But these commonplace complications weren't what set M/C Wilson apart from the other preemies who inhabited the neonatal intensive care unit that December of 1977; what made this baby different from the others was a freak mechanical failure, a unique high-tech disaster that occurred on the boy's sixth night of life.

Among the usual NICU paraphernalia to which M/C Wilson was attached as he lay on his warming table mattress were the ventilator, the bili lights, the umbilical artery catheter with its mechanical fluid delivery pump, and the cardiac monitor with its three chest leads that were pasted onto the infant's skin. Besides these devices there was a temperature control feedback loop, an ingenious device composed of a temperature sensor, a tiny needle stuck through the superficial portion of the infant's skin and connected by a wire to a thermostat that measured the child's temperature and, depending on the reading, either activated the heater built into the canopy of the warming table or switched the heater off. When working properly, the temperature control feedback loop provided a safeguard against drastic, rapid drops or elevations in the infant's body temperature resulting from immaturity of the central nervous system. When working improperly, however, the apparatus could become a serious threat to life and limb.

Sometime during M/C Wilson's sixth night, the temperature sensor that had been embedded into the skin of the baby's chest stopped functioning. The thermostat, mistakenly monitoring a low reading from the crippled sensor, kept the warming table's heating mechanism going full blast. By the time anyone happened to notice, at around four o'clock that morning, M/C Wilson was literally roasting; using a conventional glass thermometer, the nurse who made the discovery measured the baby's temperature at 106 degrees. It was undoubtedly much higher than that, but 106 was the highest reading registered on that type of thermometer.

On discovering this horrible screw-up, the nurse acted quickly. She immediately moved the child to a new warming table whose heating unit was off. After switching the beds, she next removed all the infant's clothing, exposing his body to the much cooler ambient temperature of the NICU. Then she rushed down the hall to the on-call room, awakened the intern and resident who were on that night, and reported the incident to them.

Telling the house officers what had happened yielded only the most minimal of helpful results. Not surprisingly, neither Jennifer White, the intern who was on call that night, nor Jeff Goodman, the cross-covering senior resident who was also present, had ever had any experience caring for a patient who'd been baked like a Thanksgiving turkey. Not having a clue as to what should be done for this unfortunate child, Jeff immediately called Jonathan Simon, the neonatologist in charge of the NICU, at home to ask for advice. Dr. Simon, who himself had never been faced with a situation quite like this and, likewise, had no idea what needed to be done, made a few tentative suggestions. For one, he ordered Jeff to turn up the rate at which the IV fluid was running. Second, figuring that too rapid cooling would probably make the baby's condition worse, he told Jeff to make sure the kid's temperature came down slowly. But those were the only suggestions the attending could offer; those, and the instructions that everybody watch the baby very closely over the next forty-eight hours and offer as much supportive care as possible.

And watch M/C Wilson we did. After that night ended and the day staff arrived for work, we all looked on as, during the early morning hours of the baby's seventh day, M/C Wilson's body temperature drifted back into the normal range. We watched as his temperature continued to dip ever lower, below 99 degrees, then below 98. Finally, when it went just below 97 degrees at a little after ten o'clock the next morning, Dr. Simon ordered that the heating unit on the warming table be switched on. Then, with the temperature now stabilized, we watched as the baby's anterior fontanelle, the soft spot on the top of the skull, became full and began to bulge, a sign of increasing pressure within the baby's brain; we looked on as the child's head circumference increased by two full centimeters during a four-hour period and his level of activity decreased, so that it appeared as if he'd fallen into coma. "That's it," Jonathan Simon finally concluded when a measurement of the infant's head circumference during the late afternoon showed that the size was still increasing. "The kid must have had a mammoth intracranial hemorrhage. He's dead. We might as well stop everything we're doing."

But that wasn't what the child's mother wanted us to do. In discussions with her on the day after the incident occurred and in the days that followed, Dr. Simon laid out the worst. During the first meeting, at about four o'clock on the afternoon of M/C Wilson's seventh day of life, the neonatologist apologized profusely to Ms. Wilson. Sitting in his small office, the attending explained in detail exactly what had happened. Bowing his head slightly, he said, "What happened to your baby was a horrible accident, a real tragedy, and the staff and I are all terribly sorry about it. Things like this should never, ever happen in a hospital in a city like New York."

The mother, who had been crying all through Dr. Simon's account of the incident, then asked the neonatalogist if he thought the baby was permanently harmed. "Unfortunately, I'm pretty sure he is," Dr. Simon replied. "It looks to me as if the baby's suffered a major intracranial hemorrhage; that means that he's had some bleeding into the substance of his brain, the same kind of thing that happens when older people have a stroke. Only I think the baby's stroke was much worse than most. I'm afraid the bleeding has probably caused serious and permanent damage to his brain."

The woman's crying grew louder; other than the sound of her sobbing, the room became quiet for a short while. "How sure are you?" she finally managed to ask.

"I'm sorry to say that I'm almost positive," the attending said. "The baby's soft spot has started to bulge, and his head circumference, the size of his head, has grown very rapidly over the last few hours; those are usually signs that something other than brain is occupying the skull, something like blood. And his activity today is very depressed; it's as if he's in a coma. There's no way to be a hundred percent sure," he concluded, "but if I had to bet on it, I'd say that the baby has suffered a very serious intracranial hemorrhage."

And that ended the first meeting. Over the course of the next forty-eight hours, as the baby's head circumference continued to increase and his activity level remained depressed, the attending gently suggested to the woman that we begin to withdraw some of the extraordinary means that were being used to keep M/C Wilson alive. "He's showing no signs of waking up," Dr. Simon told her. "I'm afraid that keeping him on the ventilator is only delaying the inevitable."

But Ms. Wilson resisted each attempt to get her to allow her son to die. "I don't believe he's as bad as you all say he is," she told us during work rounds on the morning of M/C Wilson's ninth day. "I think he's going to make it."

"I hope you're right," Dr. Simon replied.

Because as a fourth-year medical student I could do very little to help either M/C Wilson or any of the other babies inhabiting the NICU, I became a kind of ombudsman during the next few days, carrying messages between Ms. Wilson and the medical staff. On most days I spoke with the woman three or four times, bringing her medical bulletins from the staff and keeping her up to date on her son's condition. After I finished my report, the boy's mother would rattle off a series of questions about her son's condition. Most of the time I had absolutely no idea how to answer these questions, but I always promised Ms. Wilson that I'd ask Dr. Simon and report back to her with his response. Once I got answers from the attending I'd return to talk with the woman, playing a kind of medical telephone game.

Things went on like that for about a week, until my month's rotation came to an end and I left the NICU. Since I didn't hear again of M/C Wilson or his mother, I assumed that the child died soon after the beginning of the new year. And now, amazingly, I was watching him sit in that examining room, looking and acting like a normal three-and-a-half-year-old. "Albert is the baby

who got heated up to a hundred and six degrees?'' I
asked, flabbergasted.

The mother simply nodded her head.

''When did he—how long did he stay in the hospital?''
I asked, still awestruck.

''Three and a half months,'' the woman said. Then
she began to tell me the incredible story. Albert had remained comatose, his anterior fontanelle bulging, his entire head swollen, for nearly a week. But then, gradually,
over the course of the next week, the baby's symptoms
simply resolved. First he started moving around again,
shifting his arms and legs the way he had before he'd
been baked; then his fontanelle became softer and flatter,
and with the generalized decrease in swelling the boy's
head circumference shrunk to a more normal size.

Jonathan Simon ultimately concluded that Albert had
not suffered an intracranial hemorrhage, as he'd originally thought. Rather, as a result of excessive hyperther-
mia (elevation of temperature), he had developed severe
cerebral edema, or swelling of the brain. The presence
of the soft spot in the baby's skull saved the child's life;
the fontanelle provided a kind of escape hatch, a safety
valve that allowed the brain to swell outward without
causing any serious damage. Once the swelling of his
brain had resolved, apparently on its own, Albert, none
the worse for wear, rallied.

Over the weeks following his recovery from hyper-
thermia, the baby's systems gradually matured. By the
time he was six weeks old his lungs had healed and he'd
outgrown his need for the mechanical ventilator. By two
months M/C Wilson remained in the hospital only because he still weighed less than five pounds, the required
weight for discharge from the NICU. He spent another
month and a half at Jonas Bronck as a grower and was
finally discharged home at three and a half months.

''It sounds like a miracle,'' I said after Ms. Wilson
finished telling me the story.

''It is a miracle,'' the woman said emphatically. ''First
all of you doctors told me my baby was going to die.

Then when he didn't die, you all said he was going to be badly brain damaged. I never believed any of it, not even for a minute. I knew all along that my Albert was going to be all right; I was sure my boy would get out of the hospital and wind up normal. I knew it, because I prayed to God. I had faith in Him, and He helped my boy; He helped Albert in ways no doctor ever could.''

Not able to think of a response, I simply nodded. After thanking me for my help, Ms. Wilson put the prescription I had given her into her pocketbook and lifted her miracle son off her lap. Together they headed for the door.

It was after midnight; the night float had arrived, and my shift had come to an end at last. But rather than running for the door and heading home, I sat in the empty examining room for a while. I thought about M/C Wilson and what his mother had said. Through four years of medical school, through a year of internship and two more of residency, I'd come to see clearly how limited medicine and the physicians who practiced it were. The things that happened to people, the medical ailments that afflicted them, were either simple and easily treated or so complex and critical that their outcomes were virtually out of our hands. In a case like that of M/C Wilson, through forces that none of us understood, the patient would either get better or die. I realized that Ms. Wilson was probably right: maybe it was all up to God.

Still thinking of that little boy and his mother, I packed up my instruments, threw my pack on my back, and headed out of the quiet hospital toward the parking lot.

Epilogue

We enter medical school filled with idealism and compassion. We physicians come to the field of medicine because we have the desire to do something with our lives that will help others, and what happens to us? We spend two years sitting in lecture halls, listening to scientists who most of the time would much rather be off in their labs carrying out their research than lecturing to a group of future doctors. We learn biochemistry, histology, anatomy, cell biology, physiology, and pathology—hard, cold sciences that have to do with the functioning of the human body and the etiology of human diseases, but which lack that key element all of us crave: contact with living, breathing patients. And when those first two years of medical school come to an end and we're at last unleashed on real patients, we wind up spending the bulk of our time learning the techniques of patient care, the nuts and bolts of medical practice, from interns and residents. Many of these house officers, who just a few years before were themselves medical students, have, through a combination of exhaustion, a consequence of spending every third or fourth night on call in the hospital without any sleep, and depression, the cumulative result of all the miseries with which they must deal on a daily basis, become jaded, bitter, and angry—angry at the hospital for demanding that they work so hard, and angry at the patients, whom they come to view as their natural enemies, depriving them of the chance to lead anything resembling a normal life. As third- and fourth-year medical students, we watch the interns and residents work endlessly during their nights on call, we listen when they wish their patients would die so they can get a few extra hours of sleep, and we shake our heads in disbelief and swear that no matter what happens, no matter how intolerable things become, we'll make it our business never, ever to feel that way about any of our own patients.

Then we ourselves become interns. We're forced to work those same hours and to watch our own patients grow sick and die, and suddenly we realize that the promise we made to ourselves late at night during our third year of medical school is one we're not going to be able to keep. I was less than two months into my internship when, while trying to start an intravenous line on a baby who seemed to have no veins, I found myself jabbing needles over and over again into the child's skin, attempting to inflict pain and suffering on the infant, for no reason other than the fact that he was keeping me from getting to bed. The situation only becomes worse during residency when, as a result of the accumulation of all these factors, we find ourselves becoming numb, working like automatons, accomplishing what needs to be done with a minimum of emotional engagement. By the end of our training, not only do we no longer have the desire to help others, we don't want to be bothered by anyone. Most graduating senior residents would choose to move to some deserted South Sea island if they only could, to live out the rest of their lives as virtual hermits.

Medical education in the United States today takes people who enter the system filled with humanism and idealism and ultimately forces them to surrender these ideals by the very process that turns them into technically competent and intellectually capable physicians. Even the medical educators who support the system, those who believe that interns and residents, in order to become good physicians, must work a hundred or more hours a week with shifts lasting thirty-six hours at a stretch, acknowledge that this schedule may temporarily obliterate the good qualities medical students bring with them. But they also argue that physicians' desire to help their fellow man quickly returns once the training process is completed. This argument may be true in many cases, but it certainly isn't true in every case. Plenty of physicians practicing today care little about anything other than their own incomes and life-styles. These doctors are responsible for the image of the uncaring, unfeeling, money-grubbing physician in the minds of many Americans.

None of this makes any sense. Humanism and idealism are qualities we should demand in our physicians, qualities we should be building on, not destroying as a consequence of the training process. Producing physicians who see their primary job as serving mankind is possible, but accomplishing this goal will take major changes in the current system of medical education.

These changes must begin even before the start of medical school with the selection of candidates who will, with the proper training, blossom into caring, concerned physicians. Admissions committees at schools throughout the United States are charged with choosing entering classes from among thousands of applicants. Because so many persons seek to become physicians, applicants with the most outstanding objective records—the highest undergraduate grade point averages, the best scores on the Medical College Aptitude Test—are preferred. Although these high-achieving applicants often excel in the basic science courses offered in the first two years of medical school, their academic performance provides no guarantee, nor any real reason to believe, that they will prove to be competent and caring physicians. Medical school admissions committees must not settle simply for academic excellence; they must take the time to select applicants who, in addition to having capable minds, will make compassionate and sensitive doctors. Searching for these qualities, which are after all far more subjective than college grades and board scores and therefore much

more difficult to identify, will ensure the high caliber of
our future physicians.

But even compassionate and sensitive medical students
become bored and jaded when they are subjected to the
traditional system of medical education. For instance, the
first two years of medical school have traditionally been
spent in lecture halls and laboratories. Although a mas-
tery of the basic sciences is unquestionably important for
would-be physicians, sitting in a classroom, listening to
lectures for two full years when what one really wants to
be doing is caring for patients will take its toll. Patient
care experiences should be incorporated into the first two
years of medical school.

Some steps have already been taken to institute this
change. A few years ago, for instance, our medical school
began a new course called Introduction to Clinical Medicine. Running through the curriculum of the entire first
and second years, ICM brings fledgling students into
contact with real patients; through weekly exercises, future physicians interview and examine individuals with a
multitude of afflictions, including end-stage cancer and
heart disease, AIDS, and diabetes. Students learn first-
hand what life is like for persons with chronic diseases,
and they come to understand the effect of long-term illnesses not only on patients but also on patients' families.
ICM, which should serve as a model for similar courses
at every medical school in the country, has been a re-
sounding success. Nearly all the sutdents have benefited
from the experience, and the patients who have been involved have appreciated the opportunity to express to the
young doctors in training their gripes and complaints
about the medical care delivery system. Moreover, members of the clinical faculty have found that students seem
better prepared for their initial experiences with hospitalized patients during the clinical clerkships that compose the third year of school.

But first- and second-year courses such as ICM are not
nearly enough. In addition to preparing students for their
work on the wards before the start of their third year,

ongoing support must be continued through the final two clinical years of medical school.

During a typical on-call day, third-year medical students spend two or three hours in didactic sessions with attending physicians, the faculty members employed jointly by hospitals and medical schools who make daily ward rounds, conduct conferences, and give lectures. For the rest of the day, however, an additional twenty-one or twenty-two hours, each student works alone with an intern or resident. The vast bulk of the teaching of clinical medicine thus falls to these house officers, the overworked, overtired, overstressed young doctors on whose shoulders most patient care responsibilities rest. Not only do students learn basic skills and patient management techniques from interns and residents, they can't help but be influenced by the attitudes of these recent medical school graduates. Clinical clerks learn how to draw blood, start IVs, write nurses' orders and admission notes, and plan patients' discharges, but they also pick up the derogatory slang terms for particularly difficult or unpleasant patients which interns and residents use almost automatically, such as GOMER (an acronym for Get Out of My Emergency Room), GORK (for God Only Really Knows, used to describe patients who have suffered serious neurological damage), and SHPOS (for Sub-Human Piece of Shit). Although such slang can reflect the kind of gallows humor necessary to get through the dire situations that often arise in hospitals, medical students too readily come to accept the callous sensibility underlying these terms.

One solution to this less-than-optimal situation is to uncouple medical students from the house officers, a mating that was initially created out of necessity. If students were assigned to attending physicians rather than to interns, two goals would be accomplished: first, unburdening house officers of their teaching responsibilities would give interns more time to complete their work, allowing them to spend less time in the hospital; second, students matched with attending physicians would learn more from experienced doctors with, presumably, far better attitudes. Although implementing this proposal would be expensive, the long-term benefits of instilling a positive orientation toward the practice of medicine would make the investment of time and money well worth it.

Next, it is astounding that virtually no formal forum now exists during medical school and residency training for discussing the humanistic aspects of medicine. Students are taught how to diagnose and treat specific diseases, but they're never taught the methods that should be used when talking with patients who have those diseases or with their families. Little attention is paid to vitally important issues in a doctor's life, such as how to inform a patient that he has a life-threatening illness, how to care for a patient whom the physician dislikes, or what to do when confronted with a colleague who abuses drugs or alcohol. Physicians currently learn how to deal with these issues through trial and error. But in order to ensure that our doctors are successful in caring for their patients, we must not overlook such topics. We need to develop forums for continuing dialogue concerning the human and emotional aspects of patient care. Beginning in the third year of medical school, such formal programs would run through the rest of a doctor's training, including internship and residency. Like biochemistry, physiology, and pathology, this area must be made a mandatory part of medical education.

Finally, the most psychologically damaging part of medical education in the United States today is, undoubtedly, the enforced life-style of our interns and residents. House officers are often scheduled to work more than a hundred hours a week, with shifts lasting up to thirty-six hours every third or fourth day. The constant work and the chronic lack of sleep adversely affect young doctors' bodies as well as their minds. This system is grossly unfair not only to interns and residents but also, and more important, to their patients, who should be cared for by physicians whose sense and judgment have not been impaired by chronic, unrelenting exhaustion. There is no reason why this practice should continue.

In July 1988, New York became the first state to limit the number of hours house officers are permitted to work. By state mandate, no intern or resident is allowed to spend more than eighty hours a week in the hospital and no more than twenty-four hours continuously as part of a single shift. The fact that these schedule limitations had to be mandated by the state legislature is telling: the medical establishment is currently unwilling or unable to reform these antiquated and dangerous training methods.

The New York law is, I hope, only a beginning. In the future, the hours interns and residents work should shrink. Perhaps in the first part of the twenty-first century physicians will be able to look back and recall these bad old days as factory workers remember the days of the sweatshops of the early twentieth century. Unfortunately, the comparison is not exaggerated.

These recommendations offer only the beginning of what must be a long and complicated process of reforming medical education. There's no question that such changes are necessary: my experiences, and those of my colleagues, are evidence that the revolution is long overdue.